COPING WITH

HEAD INJURY

*This book is dedicated to the victims
of head injury, their families, and
the professionals who work with them
so that better understanding is possible.*

COPING WITH ────────
HEAD INJURY

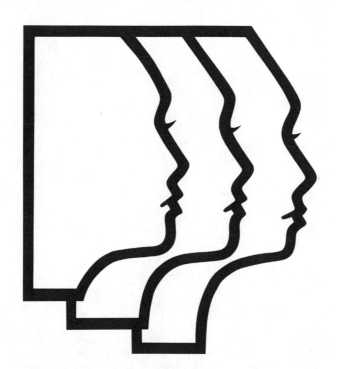

BEVERLY SLATER

with Maria Kendricken, BS, RPT and
Barbara Zoltan, MA, OTR

SLACK Incorporated, 6900 Grove Road, Thorofare, New Jersey 08086

Printed in the United States of America

Library of Congress Catalog Card Number: 88-43322

ISBN: 1-55642-078-1

Published by: SLACK Incorporated
               6900 Grove Rd.
               Thorofare, NJ 08086

Last digit is print number: 10   9   8   7   6   5   4   3   2   1

Contents

Publisher's Note

In February 1980 Beverly Slater was brought into the emergency room of a large teaching hospital, the victim of a motor vehicle accident. She had sustained head trauma, including a basilar skull fracture, and was comatose, responding only to deep pain stimulation. She was weaned from the respirator on the fourth hospital day, but her response was slow. Recovery of mentation was slow, and all memory of distant past and near past events was gone. She did not recognize family members. Concurrently she was suffering from staphylococcal pneumonia and was under therapy for that condition.

By the tenth hospital day she was fully ambulatory but still confused. On the fifteenth hospital day her mental clarity improved, and a computed tomographic scan showed evidence of cerebral contusions, both frontal and occipital. Steroid therapy was used in the post-trauma course. She was discharged to go home under the care of an attending practical nurse on the forty-sixth hospital day.

Contributors

Maria Kendricken, BS, RPT
Physical Therapy Supervisor, Head Injury Unit
New England Rehabilitation Hospital
Woburn, Massachusetts

Barbara Zoltan, MA, OTR
Lecturer, San Jose State University
Consultant, Saratoga University
San Jose, California

Acknowledgements

My thanks to my husband Harold for his support, to Mae Faltenbacher and George Barton for their encouragement in the beginning, to Loretta Tiger for her help in gathering families for interviews, to Hugh Carberry, PhD for his network support, and to the patients and families who responded to surveys about head injury.

My special gratitude to Sherri Price for the generous gift of her time and talent in writing assistance. My thanks to the staff at SLACK Incorporated, especially to Judith Paquet for providing support and direction. Her warmth and sense of humor was a tonic.

Beverly Slater

Special thanks to Mary Evans, RPT and Cheryl Kaitz, BS, RPT, specialists in head trauma rehabilitation at New England Rehabilitation Hospital, for their contributions to the physical therapy comments.

Maria Kendricken

Introduction: Awakening

Each year 700,000 people are hospitalized with some degree of head injury. Approximately 140,000 of them do not survive, according to the National Head Injury Foundation in Framingham, Massachusetts. With over 70,000 people surviving severe head trauma every year, why is so little known about it? This book is not meant to criticize but to educate. The voice of head trauma victims has been silent until now. Even the press has dubbed it "the silent epidemic." Therefore, the medical world can make judgments only on the basis of what is seen and how families react. As a victim of head trauma, I feel that I have "paid my dues" to be able to write this book and share the mistakes, triumphs, and insights I have gained in the intervening years.

It is easy to point out mistakes. It would be a simple thing to condemn with glowing examples all the misjudgments, mistreatments, false hope, or unnecessary fears. That would serve no useful purpose. I am not a neurosurgeon or a therapist. My credentials are simple: I've been there! Can an obstetrician who is not a parent effectively describe what childbirth is like? Can a comparison be drawn by someone who has never felt the pain and joy of bringing a new life into the world? Likewise, no one really knows the head trauma victim as well as the victim himself. Only recently have such patients and their families begun to form support groups to share experiences, pain, and encouragement. Until now, however, the speakers have always been doctors, rehabilitation therapists, and counselors. Doctors can merely describe symptoms; they cannot feel them. Therefore, all the literature that has been written so far is really speculation, not fact. Now is the time for the "silent" victim to speak up.

Being brain damaged is like being on the outside looking in. Imagine the frustration of being on the other side, looking out at the real world and trying to be understood. It is best described as being in a "twilight zone" — halfway in and halfway out. We may look and act "normal," but the mind does not think as a "normal" mind does. Worst of all is the emotional devastation when the victim of head trauma begins to remember his past. He recalls what he was able to do once but must learn to adjust when he realizes that he will not be the same again.

I am reminded of a "handicap" of my own. As a result of my accident, the olfactory nerves in my head were damaged. Consequently I can neither smell nor taste. All foods taste the same, except for texture and temperature. My enjoyment of food is limited because of these restrictions, and as a result food is not important to me. I eat what everyone else eats so as not to seem out of place. However, I have no recollection of what foods taste like. I do not miss the experience. Imagine how frustrating it would be if I did remember and could never again enjoy those delicious flavors! It is not difficult to imagine that you cannot smell or taste, but the process of thinking and understanding is entirely different. One of the keys in dealing with this problem is to retrain the patient to accept his limitations and develop to the limits of his capacity. Acceptance is important if the patient wants to recover.

I am living proof that there is hope for the head trauma victim. Everyone should have the opportunity to reach his potential, to become a viable human being. Some will progress more than others, and unfortunately some will not progress at all; but we should not give up hope at the first sign of failure. We must instill determination in the relatives, friends, and professional personnel involved to create a positive environment for the patient. Today many "explanations" are offered in an effort to answer what are seemingly unanswerable questions. Nonetheless, presently available treatment does not effectively satisfy the total needs of the patient.

Not long ago a lawyer jogging on the side of the road was struck by a truck. His frantic wife waited outside the intensive care unit of the hospital until the doctor came out. "I'm afraid he'll never practice law again," he said. How wrong he could be! It is true that the lawyer may never practice law again, but how can the doctor possibly know that? Everyone told my husband to put me into an institution, that I'd never be normal. Thus I suppose it is not "normal" to have written and had published two books already, or to have one of those books made into a television movie.

1

The Need
for Information

When a friend asked me how I happened to be writing this book, I truthfully answered, "Because I'm crazy!" We laughed about it, but I really did think that it was a crazy idea. Not until people started to listen and ask questions did the idea begin to take on a new aspect — that of the possible. Four years after my accident I realized that the number of cases of head trauma was increasing every year.

I was invited to lecture before a head trauma support group, and after speaking of my experiences, I invited questions or comments. Pandemonium nearly broke out. Members of the audience were like thirsty survivors in a desert, eager for information. Everyone there was a parent or spouse of a head trauma victim. When I asked about sources of information about head trauma, they all responded that there was almost nothing available. The only literature written about head trauma consisted of pamphlets and newsletters with articles by neurosurgeons and psychiatrists, but there was not one article by a victim.

Every month I went to these meetings. I became acquainted with the leaders of support groups in New Jersey, Pennsylvania, and Massachusetts. They encouraged me to search for information about head trauma, but there was little or nothing to be found. Statistics were startling when it came to head injuries in the United States alone. Some said that there were 1.5 million cases known; others said that there were 70,000 each year. Regardless of which figure is accurate, it is still a phenomenal number. To think that such a large group has been virtually unheard of is unbelievable.

Information must be made available, not only for the therapists and professional people dealing with victims of head trauma, but also for the bewildered families who do not know where to turn for help. My experiences as related in my first book, /Stranger in My Bed,/ evoked such a reaction that I felt compelled to do something about this tragedy.

According to the 1980 Surgeon General's report, "Trauma is the leading cause of death in the United States for persons under the age of 34." Information obtained from the National Head Injury Foundation, Inc., in Framingham, Massachusetts, reveals that the number of deaths each year from trauma to the head is estimated at over 100,000. The estimated prevalence of head injuries in the United States is 1.0 to 1.8 million. Even more staggering is the fact that the 50,000 people a year who survive serious head injuries sustain intellectual impairment sufficient to preclude their return to a normal life.

The National Head Injury Foundation just mentioned has a mailing list of 44,438. Families and health care professionals are on the list, of course, but imagine the enormous number of other people who get no information about head injury but are suffering with it or are related to someone who is. However, it looks as if this mailing list will continue to grow because in 1980 there were only 15 head injury programs and in 1985 there were 500. As word spreads, the numbers increase.

There are approximately 10,000 head injury health care professionals (including physicians) in this country. Of these, 4000 are associated with this foundation. One wonders about the other 6000 and how they are obtaining information.

Recently the Task Force on Head Injury of the American Congress on Rehabilitation Medicine distributed 5000 copies of a survey, the names being taken from National Head Injury Foundation lists. I was appalled to learn that only 426 responses were received. Why? My guess is that there was a lack of information or disregard of the urgency in returning the survey forms. Could this small amount, less than 10 per cent of the total, yield statistics representative of the entire group? On a larger scale, I realized that the sample group to whom the survey forms were sent represented less than 10 per cent of the national figure for the number of head injuries in one year alone. In other words, the responses to the survey came from less than 1 per cent of that total, and only a fraction of the entire head injured population.

Of the 426 responses received, half were from members (patients and families). The remainder came from physicians, therapists, nurses, and other specialists or administrators. To emphasize what is lacking today, a majority of the professionals felt that there was definitely something missing; their needs, and the needs of their patients, were not being met. Almost all the professionals felt that there should be a professional newsletter spanning all the disciplines. No such thing is available as yet.

Statistics can only go so far in relating facts and opinions. I could easily prepare a pamphlet with graphs and other statistical information, but what purpose would it serve? I felt that the only way to adequately approach the questions relating to head trauma was by direct contact — interviews, questionnaires, seminars, and discussion groups. Visiting a variety of rehabilitation hospitals and centers and speaking to staff members acquainted me with both sides of the issue. I was now an outsider trying to present an unbiased view as well as an insider with first hand experience in the field.

The first step in this massive undertaking was to use the statistics I had gathered to provide basic background information for the reader, whether a family member, a victim, a therapist, or another member of a related professional field. Because many families complained that too much information being provided was useless or invalid, I felt it important to sift through everything presently available and compile my findings in one readable and informative source as a basis for my positive approach to the treatment of head injury.

I have learned that most of these injuries occur in people under the age of 30, and most are injured as a result of tragic motor vehicle or sports accidents. Other causes include falls, assaults, gunshot wounds, diving accidents, being struck by tree limbs, bicycle accidents, child abuse, horseback riding, plane crashes, and lightning accidents. Almost 70 per cent, however, are in some way motor vehicle related (including motorcycle accidents). Head trauma may strike regardless of race, creed, or religion; it is an "equal opportunity" disease, which is avoidable in most cases. In view of the large number of people affected, it is hard to believe how little has been done.

From the layman's point of view it seems that a little care could avoid much tragedy. Fortunately drunk driving laws are becoming stricter, but there are many avoidable accidents that do not involve alcohol. More caution could have prevented some. Parents, particularly, must teach their children to be careful when crossing streets or riding bicycles. Good drivers know that one must drive defensively and wear seat belts. It takes only a fraction of a second to change a life completely as well as affect the lives of many others.

In view of the large number of people affected, it is difficult to believe how little has been done in regard to head injury. Since there will probably never be a way to totally eliminate this tragedy, help must be made available. For the families and professionals who attend these unfortunate people, I want to present a guide, a roadmap to understanding and treating head trauma victims. It is time for a new "awakening," both for the victims and for those caring for them.

We must have a clear picture of the consequences of head trauma before proceeding further. According to the New Jersey Head Injury Association, Inc., in Edison, a serious head injury usually results in loss of consciousness or coma, which may be brief, lasting only a few minutes, or may continue for days or weeks. If the period of coma is brief, recovery to full or nearly full function is likely; as the time in coma lengthens, intellectual and speech impairment, behavioral disorders, and related physical disabilties can become problems. The individual and his family face a prolonged period of rehabilitation that can last for years. Although most head injuries result from accidents, similar problems can result from encephalitis, a reduction in the supply of oxygen to the brain, cerebral hemorrhage, and cerebrovascular accident.

It is important to identify the characteristics of the head injured individual in more detail so that family members and professionals can better deal with the patient's treatment. Not all such victims suffer the physical, mental, and personality changes to be mentioned. The results depend on many factors, particularly the preinjury personality and learning style, the location and severity of the injury, the time that has elapsed since the injury, and the patient's psychological reaction to the injury.

From the Head-Injury Services of the Brown Schools (a system of psychiatric hospitals, group homes, and transitional living centers located in various states) the following characteristics are enumerated:

1. Motor deficits. Such deficits include paralysis (partial or total), poor balance, decreased endurance, loss of the ability to plan motor movements (apraxia), poor coordination (ataxia), and stiffness (spasticity). Orthopedic involvement (fractured bones, sprained or strained muscles and ligaments) is very common, as is the development of increased bone growth in the joint itself (heterotrophic bone), which affects joint mobility at the shoulders, elbows, hips, and knees.

Response:

Additional motor deficits can include rigidity, abnormal movement patterns or decreased isolated control, poor integration of primitive reflexes, and associated reactions.

—Barbara Zoltan, MA, OTR

2. Sensory deficits. All sensory systems may be affected. The deficit may involve either a decrease or an increase in sensitivity to touch, smell, sound, and movement. These deficits affect the patient's ability to perceive his body and environment. For example, a person may neglect one side of his body, or be unable to judge distances, sort our geometric shapes, distinguish right from left, or find his way around a building or area.

Response:

The author has touched on an important area of deficits, that of perceptual deficits. In addition to sensory, motor, cognitive, visual, and behavioral deficits, the patient may exhibit perceptual deficits such as impaired form, size, depth, and figure ground perception, as well as decreased spatial relations or position in space, part-whole integration, and constructional apraxia. For detailed information on these and other perceptual deficits, the reader is referred to the references.[1]

—Barbara Zoltan

3. Visual deficits. Deficits in gross visual skills may include lack of visual attention, decrease in oculomotor skills (visual scanning and saccadic eye movements), problems with visual fields, and visual neglect.

4. Speech and language deficits. The patient may not be able to understand what is said, or he may not be able to make himself understood (aphasia), or he may have difficulty in recalling words and names (anomia) or in articulating words (dysarthria).

5. Cognitive deficits. These deficits include disorientation (who one is, where one is, the current time, and those around one), attention deficits (the patient cannot focus on a task without being distracted), concentration, memory, judgment, problem solving, switching from one topic to another, meaningless repetition, inflexibility (in adapting to changes in routine), and the ability to understand abstract ideas. This type of deficit is the most difficult one for family members and friends to accept. The cognitive changes cannot be "seen" easily, and the patient's limitations are unexpected. 6. Denial. The patient may not be aware of his current situation, possibly because of actual damage to the brain or his reaction to the injury. On a physical level, a patient may continually try to get up when he is actually unable to stand. On a cognitive level he may appear to be functioning well, but his judgment is impaired. He may wish to return to work when, in fact, he is unable to carry out the tasks of his job.

7. Regulatory disturbances. A patient may be easily fatigued, his sleeping patterns may change, and he may not be able to sit through lengthy sessions of therapy. He may lose bowel and bladder control, body temperature control, and control of his consumption of foods and liquids.

8. Personality changes. Apathy, rapid changes in emotion, irritability, depression, and a lack of initiative are common. The patient may become impulsive, aggressive and abusive, and easily frustrated. He may be sexually impulsive or have a decreased sex drive. He may also be socially immature, exhibiting silly and childlike behavior.

9. Traumatic epilepsy. Two types of seizures may occur. One is the major motor or "generalized seizure"; the patient may begin making rapid body movements, lose consciousness, lose bowel and bladder control, and breathe irregularly. He may regain consciousness quickly, feel confused, and complain of soreness. This type of seizure often can be treated with medication. The second type, the "focal motor seizure," is characterized by odd twitching or jerking movements. The patient usually does not lose consciousness, and the seizure does not last long. Anticonvulsant medications, such as Dilantin, are often prescribed as a preventive measure.

To help the reader understand what is done in therapy I will explain the various stages of recovery typical of head trauma, as outlined by Chris Hagen, PhD, Danese Malkmus, MA, Patricia A. Durham, MS at Rancho Los Amigos Hospital in Downey, California. It is commonly accepted that there are eight levels of cognitive function, or stages of recovery.

1. No Response
Patient appears to be in a deep sleep and is completely unresponsive to any stimuli presented to him.

2. Generalized Response

Patient reacts inconsistently and nonpurposefully to stimuli in a nonspecific manner. Responses are limited in nature and are often the same regardless of stimulus presented. Responses may be physiological changes, cross body movements and vocalization. Responses are likely to be delayed. The earliest response is to deep pain.

3. Localized Response

Patient reacts specifically but inconsistently to stimuli. Responses are directly related to the type of stimulus presented, as in turning head toward a sound or focusing on an object presented. The patient may withdraw an extremity and vocalize when presented with a painful stimulus. He may follow simple commands in an inconsistent, delayed manner, such as closing his eyes, squeezing or extending an extremity. Once external stimuli are removed, he may lie quietly. He may also show a vague awareness of self and body by responding to discomfort by pulling at nasogastric tube or catheter or resisting restraints. He may show a bias toward responding to some persons, especially family and friends, but not to others.

4. Confused-Agitated

Patient is in a heightened state of activity with severely decreased ability to process information. He is detached from the present and responds primarily to his own internal confusion. Behavior is frequently bizarre and nonpurposeful relative to his immediate environment. He may cry out or scream out of proportion to stimuli even after removal, may show aggressive behavior, attempt to remove restraints or tube or crawl out of bed in a purposeful manner. He does not discriminate among persons or objects and is unable to cooperate directly with treatment efforts. Verbalization is frequently incoherent or inappropriate to the environment. Confabulation may be present; he may be hostile. Gross attention to environment is very brief and selective attention often nonexistent. Being unaware of present events, patient lacks short term recall and may be reacting to past events. He is unable to perform self-care activities without maximum assistance. If not disabled physically, he may perform automatic motor activities such as sitting, reaching and ambulating as part of his agitated state but not as a purposeful act, or upon request, necessarily.

5. Confused-Inappropriate

Patient appears alert and is able to respond to simple commands fairly consistently. However, with increased complexity of commands or lack of any external structure, responses are nonpurposeful, random or, at best, fragmented toward any desired goal. He may show agitated behavior but not on an internal basis, as in Level 4, but rather as a result of external stimuli and usually out of proportion to the stimulus. He has gross attention to the environment, is highly distractible and lacks ability to focus attention to a specific task without frequent redirection. With structure, he may be able to converse on a social-automatic level for short periods of time. Verbalization is often inappropriate; confabulation may be triggered by present events. Memory is severely impaired, with confusion of past and present in reaction to ongoing activity. Patient lacks initiation of functional tasks and often shows inappropriate use of objects without external direction. He may be able to perform previously learned tasks when structured for him but is unable to learn new information. He responds best to self, body, comfort, and often, family members. The patient can usually perform self-care activities with assistance and may accomplish feeding with supervision. Management on the unit is often a problem if the patient is physically mobile as he may wander off, either randomly or with vague intention of "going home."

6. Confused-Appropriate

Patient shows goal-directed behavior, but is dependent on external input for direction. Response to discomfort is appropriate, and he is able to tolerate unpleasant stimuli; e.g., NG tube when need is explained. He follows simple directions consistently and shows carryover for tasks he has relearned; e.g., self-care. He is at least supervised with old learning; unable to be maximally assisted for new learning with little or no carryover. Responses may be incorrect due to memory problems but are appropriate to the situation. They may be delayed to immediate and he shows decreased ability to process information with little or no anticipation or prediction of events. Past memories show more depth and detail than recent memory. The patient may show beginning awareness of his situation by realizing he doesn't know an answer. He no longer wanders and is inconsistenly oriented to time and place. Selective attention to tasks may be impaired, especially with difficult tasks and in unstructured settings, but is now functional for common daily activities. He may show vague recognition of some staff and increased awareness of self, family and basic needs.

7. Automatic-Appropriate

Patient appears appropriate and oriented within hospital and home settings, goes through daily routine automatically but robot-like, with minimal to absent confusion and has shallow recall for what he has been doing. He shows increased awareness of self, body, family, food, people and interaction in the environment. He has superficial awareness of but lacks insight into his condition, decreased judgment and problem solving and lacks realistic planning for his future. He shows carryover for new learning at a decreased rate. He requires at least minimal supervision for learning and safety purposes. He is independent in self-care activities and supervised in home and community skills for safety. With structure, he is able to initiate tasks or social and recreational activities in which he now has interest. His judgment remains impaired. Prevocational evaluation and counseling may be indicated.

8. Purposeful-Appropriate

Patient is alert and oriented, is able to recall and integrate past and recent events and is aware of and responsive to his culture. He shows carryover for new learning if acceptable to him and his life role and needs no supervision once activities are learned. Within his physical capabilities, he is independent in home and community skills. Vocational rehabilitation, to determine ability to return as a contributor to society, perhaps in a new capacity, is indicated. He may continue to show decreases relative to premorbid abilities in quality and rate of processing, abstract reasoning, tolerance for stress and judgment in emergencies or unusual circumstances. His social, emotional and intellectual capacities may contine to be a decreased level for him, but functional within society.

Response:

Although the Rancho Los Amigos Scale is an effective tool utilized by many profes-sionals, additional scales are available and widely utilized to measure or describe the head injury patient's level of recovery. At the most basic level, for instance, the patient's neurologist or neurosurgeon may describe the patient's loss of consciousness with terms such as coma, semicoma, stupor, obtundity, or full consciousness. The physicians or allied health professionals working with the patient may also utilize the Glasgow Coma Scale[2] or the Disability Rating Scale.[3] The Glasgow Coma Scale is utilized to assess the patient's level of awareness based on items related to motor responses, verbal responses, and eye opening. The Disability Rating Scale examines arousal/awareness, cognitive levels related to ability to handle self-care functions, physical dependence on others, and psychosocial adaptability for work, housework, or school.

Before leaving the area of recovery scales, I would like to emphasize that any scale utilized is limited by the areas it measures. The Rancho Scale, for instance, can be extremely effective in examining the patient's recovery from a cognitive or behavioral point of view, but provides little information on motor or perceptual recovery.

—Barbara Zoltan

We cannot predict the changes that will occur in the victim of head trauma. Why? To answer that I will briefly explain the function of the control centers of the brain. The brain is protected by a fluid, which allows it to "float" slightly within the skull. Different portions of the brain control thinking (the cortex), movement (the cerebellum), and consciousness, alertness, and basic bodily functions (the brain stem). The cortex is divided into lobes and hemispheres, each controlling a different function or skill.

Damage to the brain may occur during impact or may result from swelling or bleeding. When the head is hit with sudden force, the brain twists on the brain stem, causing loss of consciousness. If this loss of consciousness persists, the victim is considered to be in a coma. If the brain rebounds against the opposite side of the skull, further damage may be inflicted. The head injured victim usually suffers from diffuse damage as a result of this twisting and rebounding. As a result of this diffuse damage, a patient may present a complex picture of deficits. These can be identified through specific testing done by neuropsychologists, physicians, and therapists. Family input is essential in determining what areas of the patient's present personality and thinking differ from preinjury levels.

Preinjury characteristics such as impulsivity and short attention span may become exaggerated following head trauma.

When there is bleeding (hemorrhage) inside the brain, a mass of blood (hematoma) may put pressure on the brain tissue around it, causing further injury. If severe enough, this hematoma may require surgical evacuation; if not, the hematoma may be absorbed into the surrounding tissue. The flow of blood in the brain may be blocked, decreasing the supply of vital oxygen (hypoxia). Brain hypoxia may also result from cardiac or respiratory arrest, causing diffuse effects. As with injury to any body tissue, swelling (edema) may occur in the brain as a physiological response. This swelling puts pressure on the tissue (since the skull does not allow the brain to expand) and additional damage may occur. This may result in exacerbation of existing symptoms, or the addition of new symptoms.

As a function of the natural healing process, this swelling may decrease over time, allowing the patient's status to improve. Other factors which contribute to improvement in the patient's status are the healing of those parts of the brain that were only partially damaged, and the ability of undamaged areas of the brain to compensate (plasticity).

Response:

As the described natural healing process occurs and parts of the brain begin to compensate for others, status sometimes improves at a very rapid pace (in days or weeks) or at a very slow pace (over years with periods of plateau where little or no progress can be seen). Factors such as failed shunts, medications, infections, and seizures may hamper the healing process in the brain.

—Maria Kendricken, BS, RPT

Response:

As the author mentioned, secondary problems such as bleeding or hemorrhaging may occur. In addition, there may be infection or brain swelling. Some of these secondary problems will require surgical intervention.

In general, most head injuries are the result of the moving head striking a stationary surface or vice versa.[4,5] The degree of resulting damage depends on the amount of deceleration (sudden slowing of the moving head when it strikes a solid surface) or acceleration (brain movement when the stationary head is struck). An acceleration or deceleration injury usually results in diffuse damage. Damage from a penetrating injury (gunshot or knife), on the other hand, will be less diffuse. The more diffuse the injury, the more deficits the patient is likely to have. Brain injury can include compression — *pushing of tissues together,* shearing — *portions sliding over other portions, or* tension — *actual tearing apart of tissues. Damage can occur at the injury site (coup-lesion) or to the side opposite where the skull was struck (contrecoup lesion).[4]*

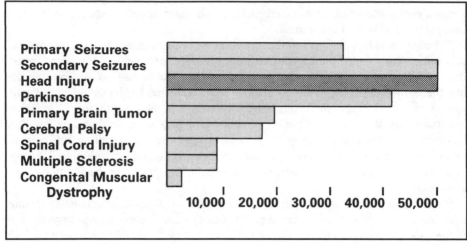

Figure 1-1.

Although the author has addressed mechanisms of brain injury, the information provided requires further clarification.

—Barbara Zoltan

Head injury is only a part of a much larger group of diseases commonly known to cause neurological dysfunction. Most common in this category is cerebrovascular disease, accounting for about 450,000 cases yearly. However, the remaining neurological diseases are reflected by statistics that are comparatively shocking. Figure 1-1 vividly shows the number of new cases of the various neurological disorders each year in comparison with head injuries.

The most startling fact revealed by these statistics is that so much is being done, and rightly so, for such illnesses as multiple sclerosis and cerebral palsy, whereas the huge population of head injured victims has no national spokesman, telethon, or public recognition. It is obvious to me that something is wrong.

Head trauma has been a problem for as long as man has existed, but until recently it did not even have a satisfactory name. The old term, "brain damaged," reflected a lack of understanding of many of the problems involved. Today new techniques in treatment are being developed, but scientists are still limited by what can be learned purely from observation. It is my hope to be a "voice" for this "silent epidemic" in order to encourage the creation of new approaches to the treatment and rehabilitation of this portion of the population.

References

1. Zoltan B, Siev E, Freishtat B: Perceptual and Cognitive Dysfunction of the Adult Stroke Patient. Thorofare, NJ, Slack, Incorporated, 1986.

2. Jennett B, Bond M: Assessment of outcome after severe brain damage. Lancet, 1975, p 480.

3. Rappaport M, et al.: Disability rating scale for severe head trauma: Coma to community. Arch Phys Med Rehabil 63 (March): 1982.

4. Jennett B: An Introducction to Neurosurgery. Ed 3. London, William Heinemann Medical Books, 1977.

5. Brain L, Walton N: Brain Diseases of the Nervous System. Ed 7. New York, Oxford University Press, 1969.

2

The Start of a New Life
Emergence After Injury

The details that led me to "start again" are public knowledge. In February 1980 I was crossing a street in Philadelphia and was struck by a turning car. I was thrown onto the car's hood, and after the car stopped I was thrown to the street and landed on my head, sustaining head trauma. I "died" twice and was revived, and then remained in a coma for several days. When I woke up, it was as though I was a newborn infant. Everything around me was new and strange. All faces were unrecognizable, and words were merely sounds. My husband, my children, my parents — all were strangers.

I was fortunate that there were no broken bones or internal injuries. I was bruised all over, but there was no physical impairment. The damage was in my brain, not my body. My amnesia was total, or what is called "long term." Forty-eight years of my life were erased in a moment.

I was a patient in the hospital for about seven or eight weeks. During that time I was cared for by many professionals: physical therapists, occupational therapists, speech therapists, recreational therapists, psychiatrists, and psychologists. Each new exposure added confusion to an already incomprehensible world. Growing up is a frightening experience in itself. Imagine going through it when you have to start close to age 50!

When I was able to breathe without a respirator and became ambulatory, I was impossible. I must have been a nurse's worst nightmare — uncooperative, abusive, and totally incoherent. The fact that I loved to explore the hospital on my own did not help matters. I did not understand what I was doing at the time, nor did I care. Like a baby, I was self-centered. Everyone was waiting eagerly for me to regain my memory, and I was tiring of their asking me repeatedly whether I remembered this or that. How could they jog my memory when I did not even know what a memory was?

"What We Have Here Is a Failure to Communicate"

Chronologically I was 48. Developmentally I had just been born. When people who knew me spoke as though I should understand, they did not realize that for me it was like hearing a foreign language for the first time. Moreover, there was a total lack of language ability because at that time I could not think; I could only feel and see.

When I first came out of the coma, there were many attempts at communication on both sides. Visitors tried to make me understand who they were, yet only as they continued to visit me did I become familiar with them. The more I saw them, the more they became recognizable. Like a child, I wanted to touch everyone. It was as though touching would make them real, would make me a part of them. I was so frustrated because I could not communicate and could not understand.

I smiled a lot, and everyone misunderstood. Remember how proud parents show their baby and say, "Look at the baby smile!" We all know that the baby is not usually consciously smiling; that is an instinctive reaction. So with head trauma victims: we smile often for no apparent reason. Also, like a child, we make few demands and are rather dreamy-eyed all the time. A newborn cries only when it is wet, hungry, or lonely. Likewise, we are relatively apathetic about everything in the world around us.

The nurses carried the burden in my initial rehabilitation. In the first couple of weeks after the accident I saw many strange faces, but they all had one thing in common: every one was Caucasian. I did not understand that they were Caucasian; I just felt that they were alike in some way. Color meant nothing to me.

One day a new nurse came in, and there was something different about her. I did not understand that she was black — only that she was different. She was confused by my seemingly incoherent babbling, although she was able to discern the word "different." At the time blood was being taken for laboratory tests and there was some blood on the bedsheet. A bolt of recognition seemed to hit the nurse, for she proceeded to prick her finger and show me her blood. She said "blood" and "same," and I repeated what she said. When I repeated this to others, no one seemed to understand my great discovery.

Another day another new face appeared. This one was different in still another way. She was Chinese. When I said "blood" and "same" to her, she was bewildered. Later she apparently spoke to the black nurse, who explained what I meant. The Chinese nurse then came in and pricked her own finger, saying "same." I got the point. In my childish way I had learned that people are really alike in many ways.

Today I remember this incident and realize that prejudice is not inborn; it is learned from others near us. A young child does not know black from white except that they are different, not better or worse. What a world we would have if we all thought in this way!

Those first two weeks were filled with confusion and fear. No one understood me at first. My jabbering was met with questioning looks and helplessness. I threw tantrums because of my frustration over not being understood. However, soon I began to recognize certain words that were repeated constantly. I parroted words, just as a toddler does, until they became part of my vocabulary.

My husband was there every day. He kept coming back, no matter how much abuse I hurled at him. My children had difficulty in accepting what had happened and kept looking for signs of recognition. If I had understood, I would not have hurt them or anyone else, but I was an ignorant baby with no conscience.

Thus my introduction to life was not the happiest. My world revolved around me. My visitors were close family members, nurses, and doctors, and more often than not I would throw tantrums to get them all to leave. However, my curiosity quickly took over, for I wanted to understand and be understood. That project was placed in the hands of professionals.

Physical Therapy

Memories flood my mind. My thoughts of the incidents at the beginning have faded and become confused. I remember some specific events but have to rely more on the recollections of others.

My earliest memory was of my first encounter with a physical therapist about two weeks after the accident. Although I had no broken bones, I had to receive physical therapy twice a day for an hour each time.

Response:
Physical Therapy is indicated for most patients, even those whose physical deficits may not be obvious. A comprehensive evaluation is done to assess more subtle problems such as coordination, endurance, balance, agility indoors and out, and motor planning.
—Maria Kendricken

That first day a stranger came over to my bed and asked me to move my leg. However, language meant little to me, and I did not understand what she was talking about, so she went away. She came back another time and gave the same directions, but I still did not understand. Finally, I was taken to another room in the hospital and laid on a foam pad on the floor The physical therapist told me to move my left leg — or perhaps it was my right leg. It did not matter; I had no idea what she was saying.

Response:

In the case of the described, the physical therapist should be aware of how cognitive, communication, and perceptual deficits will affect a patient's ability to move and follow directions. A therapist will try to elicit automatic movements first before giving direct verbal commmands. For example, instead of asking the patient to move the left leg, the therapist would indirectly gather the same information by asking the patient to roll or taking the patient through the rolling movement. The therapist would then observe how the left leg moves without actually having asked the patient to move it.

A conscientious physical therapist should never leave a head trauma patient unattended in therapy. A therapist tries many approaches to communicate with a patient. If a patient has a language problem, the therapist should extract this information from the medical record, the speech pathologist, or professional observation.

—Maria Kendricken

After a while she left the room, and not knowing what else to do, I fell asleep. When the therapist came back, she woke me and took me to my room upstairs.

At the time I had no feelings about what had happened. This person had a different face from the ones I had become used to, and she was using words that had no meaning to me. She was talking to me as the 48 year old woman she saw and did not understand that she was speaking to someone with the learning developmental level of an infant.

Now I can look back and analyze why I fell asleep. If you place a baby on its belly, it falls asleep. The therapist's words were just sounds with no meaning. Thus, when she left the room, I did what any baby would do.

Response:

Patients may be lethargic or fall asleep during therapy. The reason is not because when a baby is on its belly it falls asleep. Reasons why a patient may fall asleep include the following:

Lethargy secondary to trauma; poor endurance secondary to the deconditioning associated with prolonged bedrest or inactivity; medications used for infections, seizure control, spasticity, behavior, etc. (Appendix A); damage to the area in the brain which affects arousal and the reticular activating system; limited attention span and confusion where the patient gets bored or overstimulated; and loss of appetite or weight loss contributing to fatigue.

These patients generally do better and fall asleep less if treatment is initially kept short and breaks are given often.

—Maria Kendricken

Response:

Although the author's theory on why patients fall asleep is presented, a more accurate explanation is based on the underlying organic brain damage. The normal individual is able to receive, process, integrate, and interpret a constant stream of sensory stimulation from the environment. As a result of this process, the individual subsequently reacts or responds to his environment by moving, talking, looking, etc. We process sensations both on a conscious and unconscious level and attend to only relevant stimuli. Most of us, for instance, are able to block out a neighbor's dog barking in order to carry on a conversation. The head injury patient has impairments with the intake and processing of sensations. He is unable to distinguish what is relevant and what is not.

Using the previous example, a neighbor's dog barking and your conversation will register with equal importance. The patient essentially ends up taking in every sight, sound, and smell around him and trying to process them with an already impaired processing system. As a result, the patient's system goes into "sensory overload" similar to an overloaded electrical circuit. His system simply cannot handle any more and he "shuts down." One way this system shut down is displayed behaviorally is by the patient closing his eyes and sleeping. When the patient does this the family member or therapist should take the cue and temporarily discontinue the activity, continuing it in a less distracting environment and after the patient has rested.

Additional reasons for patients falling asleep relate to physical and physiological endurance issues which Marie describes.

—*Barbara Zoltan*

Every day the physical therapist came to talk with me. She would take me downstairs to a separate room where she would repeat instructions to me. After considerable time, and after her repetition of the words and demonstration, I succeeded in carrying out her instructions. Time after time she would raise first one of her legs and then the other. Those demonstrations, combined with the words, encouraged me to copy her. The principle of "monkey see, monkey do" took over.

After a while physical therapy became a game to me. The therapist and I would kneel on a mat facing each other with our arms folded in front of our chests. She performed the activity first, and then I would try to imitate her. She would try to push me off balance, and I would try to keep my balance. Then I would try to push her off balance, and she would try to keep her balance. She of course keep her balance more easily. I saw that her hands and arms were helping her keep her balance, but at that time I could not understand why mine were not helping me.

I was slow. Although there was no permanent injury to my body, the messages from my brain to my arms and legs did not arrive quickly. With repetition and copying her actions, it appeared that I was learning. I wasn't really; I was merely copying.

If my accident had happened in 1986 instead of in 1980, I feel that my treatment would have been much different. The therapist would have understood my learning developmental age and my capacities, for therapists have learned to deal with the mind as well as the body. The therapist would not have allowed me to go to sleep; she would have approached me initially as she would a baby, not as an adult.

How do you teach a young child to move one hand or the other or to show where his nose is? Parents play little games with their toddlers: "Where is your eye? Where is your tummybutton?" And the child points until he gets it right. Mommy and Daddy are proud; they applaud and tell him how good he is, how smart he is. Their approval is a big reward. As the child grows, he takes pride in these accomplishments, even without the praise. He no longer needs to be asked - he volunteers to show what he can do.

Thus, one of the keys to treating the victim of head trauma is to determine his learning and developmental age and design treatment accordingly. As I will show in several examples, I learned everything at this point in my therapy by repetition and copying. My therapist could not understand that I could respond only as a young child who does not yet comprehend. To her I was 48, and so I was a 48 year old who could not comprehend as far as she was concerned. She could not see that I could respond only as a young child who does not yet comprehend. At that time she could not understand why I did not respond or why I was doing what I did. The difference is subtle, but it is significant in the treatment of victims of head trauma.

Another anecdote further illustrates my point. At one time or another almost every child learns how to jump rope. We as adults assume that everyone can do it. But what happens when you give a very young child a jump rope? Does he know what to do with it? When, eventually, I was able to coordinate my body, when it was obvious that I was not physically impaired, the therapist handed me a rope. She told me to jump rope, assuming that I would know what to do. At that point I could not understand English well, and I did not know what she wanted me to do. She pointed to the rope and got no response that first day. On the second day we went back to the rope again. Finally, perhaps out of frustration, she took the rope and jumped rope herself. Watching her, I thought to myself in my childlike way, "That looks like fun!" Then I tried to do it myself. Day after day I tried to do what the therapist did. After at least a week, I was finally able to jump rope. Then, as soon as I had mastered that, we switched to another activity. Had the therapist known my developmental age, much time and effort would have been saved in her "trial and error" technique of teaching even the simplest thing.

Response:
Sometimes with a physically advanced patient who has difficulty understanding more complicated or unfamiliar activities, the therapist will introduce a familiar activity (such as jump roping or bicycling) in hopes that the patient will automatically carry out the

movement by calling on past memories and motor plans which may be intact and at the same time improve strength, endurance, balance, and coordination.

—Maria Kendricken

I once had the opportunity to watch a teacher try to show a child how to use a zipper. The child could not grasp the idea and became increasingly frustrated. However, when another child came over and demonstrated the technique, the first child picked it up right away. Children are the best teachers of each other, and the response is dramatic. Thus the therapist has to instruct at the child's level and show the patient what to do. Constant repetition — words as well as actions — is necessary in learning a particular skill.

I was lucky not to have suffered any other serious bodily injuries. Many victims of head trauma are severely restricted and need more time to get to the point at which I started. One has to correct the physical damage and concentrate on more basic body movements in such a case.

For example, a woman I have been working with is in her early twenties. Mary, discussed further in Chapter 3, was in an accident that resulted in head trauma and multiple physical injuries. She had been in a coma for three months and was sent, during that time, to a rehabilitation center in the hospital. One of her legs is still in a brace, although she is not confined to a wheelchair. She walks hesitantly and she has many speech problems.

Her first exposure to physical therapy included exercises for strengthening and to aid in controlling her arms. She could not see then, but her vision has now partially returned. Because she could not do what the therapist did, Mary's initial reaction was fear, because she could not understand what the therapist wanted her to do and was afraid of making the therapist angry — afraid of failure, all the fears of children.

Mary's experiences were recent, and the therapists are working with her on a child's level, but they still do not regard her as being quite as "young" as she really is. In other cases the victims are often perceived as being younger than their actual developmental age. Growth may occur much faster than the therapist expects, and recovery may be slowed as a result of communication failure. Sometimes a therapist acts in a condescending or patronizing manner merely because she is not attuned enough to the patient's stage of developmental growth, and the patient feels that he is being talked down to.

It is still difficult to understand what is going on in the victim's mind. Mary is unfortunate in being in a rehabilitation center where most of the other patients are either stroke victims or otherwise physically incapacitated. She associates herself with them, not with other victims of head trauma. The only other "normal" people she sees are her therapist and her family. If she could be with others like herself, she would not feel so different or so alone.

Jerry, who had been out of a coma only five days, was scheduled for two hours of physical and occupational therapy. His mother had dressed him in regular street clothes to go to his session (a practice I had also followed during my therapy). He was confined to a wheelchair, but his ability to verbalize was unimpaired. His amnesia was "short term." He could speak and remember the past, but he would forget what he did five minutes before. The occupational therapist taught Jerry to stack and unstack cones, to put marbles into holes, and to put differently colored and shaped pegs into the appropriate spaces. This was tedious and difficult for him; he rearranged the pegs many times. He seemed to enjoy these sessions, but he invariably fell asleep during physical therapy.

Here again falling asleep was an escape, or perhaps a childlike reaction to frustration or confusion. There came a time during my physical therapy when it was no longer fun. Then I purposely found places to hide. Unfortunately no one understood what I was doing. Everyone thought that I was confused and disoriented, but I knew what I was doing. I knew that I did not want to go to that room, even though I did not know the reasons. Perhaps it was because what had seemed like fun had begun to seem like a chore. There were various conflicting forces in my young mind: I wanted to please my "friends," yet I wanted to play. Picture a kindergarten or preschool classroom. The younger the child (or a class of children), the more limited the attention span. Unless the teacher varies the class activities frequently, disruption and boredom will ensue.

Thinking of Jerry, I am reminded of my own experiences in using pegs. The occupational therapist introduced me to the round peg. I now know that I was supposed to put the round peg into the round hole, but telling me then was useless. Finally the therapist showed me, told me, showed me again, and told me again. Eventually I copied her and was overjoyed at my success. Then she gave me a square peg. Of course, the square peg would not fit into the round hole, but I could not understand why. It took several more days of the therapist's doing it for me before I succeeded. Reflecting on my experience with the pegs, I know that I only did what the therapist did. I thought it was fun; it was a game. If she had tried to put the square peg into the round hole, I would have done likewise. I was not interested in the why and how; I wanted to play!

This part of my learning was fun. To me, everything was a game. If the therapist could do it, I could do it. But then she would ask me awkward questions: Did I know my name? Did I know where my room was? These things meant nothing to me. I could never seem to come up with the answers she wanted. The thought process was not working, and I could not grasp an idea, a mental concept. It was assumed that damage to my brain had made me react as I did, not that I was really a child in an adult's body. Even after two months of physical and occupational therapy, the consensus was that I should be institutionalized. If these events had happened now, it might have been different.

As a victim, I believe that one of the most important things that can be done immediately after a patient comes out of coma is to determine his learning developmental age limits. Precious time can be saved, and the recovery can be hastened dramatically, when everyone dealing with the patient is aware of what is going on in this "child's" mind.

The Team Approach

What happens when one is dealing with a patient with "short term" damage who cannot remember what he did five minutes before? David, in his early thirties, had been in a head-on car collision and suffered multiple injuries and short term amnesia (discussed further in Chapter 3). He spoke eloquently of his childhood but then forgot what he had just said. How could he learn? The answer is the same — constant repetition until it becomes second nature, a mechanical reaction. David learned how to go to the bathroom by doing it until the act became automatic. This is not a process of memorization; that is a concept we cannot understand. It is a learning experience, which eventually may lead to understanding. After much repetition, you begin to do things when just told to do them — not as a copying response. The feeling of accomplishment is so wonderful that you want to do the same thing over and over again, even after you are no longer asked to do it.

The learning process begins with repitition and mimicry in human beings. We have the capacity to feel the pleasure of success, even with the least significant act. Like a child, we look for the smallest sign of recognition — even a smile — that we have done something right. Today patients are often rewarded at first with something tangible, such as a special dessert, a piece of candy, or a flower. This technique has proved to be successful more quickly than offering no reward. Young schoolchildren take pleasure in receiving gold stars or Lifesavers as rewards, and adults respond to success in the same happy manner.

Another important aspect of this reward system is the therapist herself. When she makes an effort to communicate at the patient's level and "plays" with the patient, they become friends. Here is a pal whom you want to please and do things for. A bonding occurs that makes the patient want to succeed.

As the patient "grows up," this attachment becomes more of a parent-child relationship. However, a problem can develop if the attachment becomes too close, for the patient may not want to "perform" for anyone but one therapist. The solution is to integrate a program so well that any one of several therapists can substitute any time and continue with the same techniques. The use of many different people to work with the patient could be confusing for the young mind, but working with a few different people could be productive.

Response:
While it is true that a problem can develop if the attachment becomes too close, it is my experience that this is rare. I believe that it is both beneficial and desirable to work with the same therapist. The patient needs to establish rapport and trust (especially if he is suspicious, paranoid, or agitated), and the therapist who has dealt with a patient

previously can better measure progress (even if slight). Keeping the same therapist can result in better program planning and development, as well as consistency in responding to positive or negative behaviors. In addition, the team approach will be better executed, and families will have one contact person for each discipline.

—Maria Kendricken

Among the team members with whom the patient can work are family members, nurses, physicians (including internists, psychiatrists, and neuropsychologists), therapists (including those specializing in physical, occupational, speech, movement, and recreational therapy), vocational specialists, and social workers.

Other relationships grow and develop at the same time. I saw the same familiar faces every day: My husband always seemed to be there, as were other members of my family, therapists, and particularly the nurses. Because I was with the therapists for only a limited number of hours each day, most of the work of teaching me simple tasks was left to the nurse on duty.

For example, I have mentioned David's experience in learning how to go to the bathroom and recall my own way of learning. As soon as I was able to get out of bed, I was taken to the bathroom repeatedly. After watching the nurse and hearing the words many times, I gradually understood.

The same was true of taking a shower. I was given a towel and soap and told to take a shower, but of course I was not going to get clean that way. After many sessions in which I was put in the shower and washed by the nurse, she finally came in with me and showed me how she washed herself. Thereafter the copy-cat in me took over, and showering was no longer a problem.

Language was very difficult for me to comprehend. While I was learning English all over again, just as a child does, I did not understand the various meanings that words could have. For example, when I was told to "get out of bed," I fell to the floor. Every word was taken literally. When someone pointed to an object, I could identify it after much practice, but I was unable to grasp ideas or concepts. There is a great difference between pointing to me so that I would say my name and asking me, "What is your name?" A young child reacts in the same way. Eventually as the child grows older, he begins to understand the complexity of language, but when I was "growing up," no one understood what I was thinking.

It seems odd now, but when I came out of the coma, my first words were vulgarities. I later learned that this is common among head trauma victims. Now I know that the person I was before the accident did not use foul language. Thus it seems strange that I would use such words after the accident. Perhaps, as with a child, inhibitions do not exist; the mind is not in total control of the words that are spoken.

A toddler might think nothing of asking an obese woman, "Why are you so fat?" A three-year-old girl seeing a black woman for the first time innocently asks, "Why are you so dirty?" Not until we grow older do we think before we speak. I did not realize that I was insulting the people who loved me and can only hope that they understood that my inconsiderate words were not intentional.

Watching young children at school and at play now helps me to understand what was happening to me then. I remember that my favorite companions were my very young granddaughters. Because I thought at their developmental level, we had much in common. They were not inhibited by the restraints of adulthood, and we could get right down on the floor and play. If one applies this knowledge to therapy, it is reasonable to think that the therapist should "come down" to the child's level, literally. Face to face, eye to eye contact holds the patient's attention and creates the bonding that helps the "child" to learn.

Another important influence often comes from a close relative, particularly a mother, who can devote more time to the patient, allow her own involvement to inspire the patient to try harder, and recall childhood behavior and respond accordingly. Nancy's mother (see Chapter 3), for example, refused to accept the doctor's prognosis that Nancy would never be more than a "vegetable." She was able to move into the rehabilitation center with her daughter and did much of the teaching herself, because she refused to accept what the doctors had told her. A special education teacher who came to see Nancy understood what was happening almost immediately. She assessed Nancy's developmental age from her behavior and at that time predicted that Nancy would be able to graduate from high school.

Whether she is right is not important. What is significant is that there are options. One does not necessarily have to accept the words of professionals as gospel, nor does one have to believe in miracles to realize that there are unexplained cures and unexpected instances of progress. Each patient is different, and what works well for one could be useless for another. The decision must be left to the family of the victim, but that decision should be an informed one, based on knowledge as well as emotion. Throughout this book I wish to discuss common techniques and treatments that have proved successful in a number of cases and that will make rehabilitation more useful in preparing the patient for a new life.

I have said that therapists in earlier days were "shooting in the dark" to find successful techniques. Time was wasted weeding out what worked and what did not work. Chapter 4 is largely devoted to this subject. In Chapter 3 recent case histories demonstrate how patients have been treated by physical and occupational therapists. I will briefly describe each patient and give several examples of the therapeutic training used in their rehabilitation.

Response:
Throughout this book the author refers to learning and developmental age and suggests that head trauma patients should be approached as children. It is inaccurate to

assume that there is a correlation between a normal developing nervous system and one which has sustained a lesion and is healing. Treating the head injured patient as a child is not the method of choice in many insitions.

Many deficits associated with head trauma can manifest as childish behaviors. After a head injury a person may be very distractable and have a shortened attention span, impaired memory, or diminished awarenesss of his environment. These are all socially unacceptable behaviors. Treating patients like young children suggests a total reversal to childhood. Treatment must be geared specifically to the individual patient's cognitive, behavioral, and physical needs. which will change with differing activities in differing environments. We have found that structuring the environment to decrease distractability, giving simple instructions slowly to allow time for them to process, and changing tasks more often to hold attention are valuable and effective treatment approaches (see Appendix C).

With most head trauma patients damage is so diffuse that a patient cannot be considered to be at one specific developmental level or age. For example, a patient may be severely distractable or disinhibited (as a young child might be) yet still be able to balance a checkbook, and be motivated to do this rather than play childish games. We have found that most patients react negatively to being treated like children.

—Maria Kendricken

3

We Are Not Alone
Case Studies

David

David was the victim of an automobile accident in 1979 and sustained multiple injuries and head trauma. There were also visual problems. He required a tracheotomy. He was in a coma for two weeks and remained in the hospital for two months before being transferred to a rehabilitation unit for two months. He was treated as an outpatient for eight months more.

David did not emerge from the coma until two weeks after the accident. His mother was with him constantly, and spoke to him frequently even though she had been told that he could not hear her. Nonetheless David responded by wiggling his nose or sticking his tongue out. One must remember that this happened in 1979. Today physicians are convinced that therapy should begin even during the coma period, but David's mother figured this out by herself.

Therapy was extensive because of the degree of physical damage. David could not sit up well; his head rolled to one side. Nor could he use his legs or one arm at that time. Thus the physical therapist first had to concentrate on getting him up. He would be strapped into a chair from which, like a child, he would try to escape. His only wish was to get out of the hospital. He threw tantrums, cursed, and was obstinate.

David does not remember any of this. The head trauma caused short term disability. He can remember much from the past but has trouble remembering recent events, people, and his own thoughts. Thus I relied on his mother's recollections about this time.

Fortunately she had kept a diary of David's progress that was much more reliable than human memory.

The first physical therapy sessions were basically introductory. The therapist was trying to find out exactly what David could and could not do. The hospital where he was being treated did not offer too much in the way of rehabilitation training. Most of that began when he was transferred to a rehabilitation center. Throughout the hospitalization David's mother was there to encourage and assist. It was her presence that David credits as the reason for his recovery. In my case my husband was always there. Although my injuries were very different from David's, we shared many of the same feelings and experiences.

Just as I did not want to be restrained from roaming around the hospital, David fought to escape his physical limitations. He wriggled his way out of beds and chairs. He even maneuvered his way to a telephone and called his mother at 11 p.m. to get him out. Like a child, he wanted his own way and tried in every way possible to get it. He wet his bed and urinated against the wall to infuriate his "captors."

Response:

Often patients who have experienced head trauma are confused, impulsive, and unsafe, and may have impaired balance. They may try to get up by themselves, and may fall and hurt themselves. For their own safety poseybars or jackets are used to restrict them from getting up from wheelchair or bed (like David). Patients and families should be given explanations of this. The restriction should be removed as soon as the patient demonstrates improved safety awareness or is ablee to get up safely without falling.

Patients who are physically capable of walking but are confused or disoriented present another type of problem. This patient may wander around the hospital and get lost, may get onto an elevator and be unable to get out, or may go outdoors in an effort to get home and find himself in the midst of oncoming traffic or on a bus. In a hospital setting it is often not possible to provide one-on-one constant supervision for such a patient. Nurses must be aware at all times where these patients are. Often pictures of these patients are posted at the admitting desk, cafeteria, other nursing floors, and with the security guard. Electronic wrist bands sound a buzzer when the patient leaves the nursing unit. Exit doors to the unit sound buzzers when opened.

—Maria Kendricken

David's key asset was his ability to speak. He was obsessed with the idea that he was not going to sound like the "dummy" that everyone thought he was because he was brain damaged. He worked diligently to improve his language skills. Today, except for a slight limp, it is difficult to imagine that he ever had a problem.

Talking with David and his mother brings many thoughts to mind about my own experiences. The more I listened, the more I heard the same themes over and over again

— the childlike behavior, the need for repetition, the need for reward, the frustration, the failure of communication, the misunderstandings. Our injuries were different, but there is so much in common that we can discuss techniques that have been effective in treating both of us as well as thousands of other such victims.

David's mother brought up some especially interesting points. One had to do with family. A head trauma victim who was in the rehabilitation center at the same time as David had no family visiting him, no one from the outside coming in to help him. This young man, the victim of a motorcycle accident, grew increasingly worse, uncontrollable, and uncooperative, to the point that he had to be taken away. In all the cases I have learned of the patient does remarkably better when there is a close relative there to help, comfort, and teach.

In David's case it took a while to get through a period of total defeat. He did not want to do anything. Once that period had passed, he went into therapy with a vengeance. He did not want to be stereotyped as "brain damaged," and thus he went beyond his previous abilities to prove himself "normal."

Would David have recovered faster if his accident had happened now? Surely! As with me, precious time was wasted because of the lack of information in head trauma treatment.

David's first contact with the physical therapists involved learning how to stand up. Because he was unable to stand by himself, two people helped to support him. He wanted to give up, but they persisted. He had to lie on the floor and learn how to get up in case he ever fell. The therapists helped him a great deal because of his physical condition.

Response:
In David's case there were probably several other deficit areas that needed to be addressed, such as strength, sitting, balance, and control of more basic activities (coming to a sitting position and rolling in bed) in addition to attempting to stand. Getting up from the floor is an advanced activity which is usually not attempted early on.
—Maria Kendricken

When it came to occupational therapy, he was hindered by visual problems. He wore prism glasses for a while. He also had one arm in a splint. Therefore, hand-eye coordination was difficult to develop. He worked with electronic games as well as the same pegs I had used, but his recovery was slower, not only because of his physical disabilities but because of his attitude.

What can we learn by reading about David? First, we can see the many similarities in both our treatments. What was successful for me was also successful for him. Even though many things differed, we shared much in common. We can both benefit from analyzing the mistakes that were made and appreciating the time that was wasted with unproductive techniques.

Brian

Brian was hit by a car while riding his bicycle in October 1984. The result was a fractured tibia, right sided motor injury, brain hemorrhage, and head trauma. He was taken to a trauma center and stayed one month in the hospital and seven months in a rehabilitation unit.

Brian was 11 years old when he was struck by the car and thrown into its windshield, landing on his head. He was taken to a trauma center immediately, something unheard of when I had my accident. He was in a coma for two weeks before he opened his eyes. Although he looked past his mother, she was overjoyed because it happened to be her birthday. After this, he began to "lighten up," to slowly come out of the coma. When he was released from the hospital to go to a pediatric rehabilitation center, he could not speak or walk, but he seemed to respond by moving his head to indicate "yes" and "no." He was put into a wheelchair before he left the hospital but was virtually unresponsive. His attendants did succeed in getting him to make a sound, but the prognosis was not good. It was said that he would never be able to think as we do or to put thoughts together into sentences.

At the hospital, therapy was given and the nurses were invaluable, but therapy had to be limited to physical therapy and speech therapy because of his physical disability. The physicians admitted that they did not know what the outcome would be, but they were not totally pessimistic. They recognized their limitations. Brian was ready to move on to a rehabilitation center.

Once he was admitted to the rehabilitation center, Brian's prognosis seemed to improve. Everyone encouraged his family to be "cautiously optimistic," quite a change from the more negative attitude at the hospital. The nurses, in particular, were very helpful in keeping the outlook positive.

Today Brian has made great progress on the road to rehabilitation. When one meets him, it is obvious that there are still physical problems: He walks with a pronounced limp and his right side (face and arm) is weak, but these limitations do not seem to slow him down. He is an active 13 year old facing all the frustrations and pain of puberty. He talks with no coaxing and is eager to be the "star attraction." One important point came up in looking into Brian's case. Because the family knew nothing about head trauma, it was difficult to determine whether his behavior was the result of the accident or typical teenage behavior.

To illustrate, a friend of Brian's came to play with him. He ended up playing more with Brian's brother, who is one year older. Was the rivalry or jealousy Brian exhibited a result of the head injury? My guess is that all teenagers go through this phase with their siblings. It is difficult to identify the reasons. Everyone in the family admits that Brian is much more outspoken,. He is now forceful when he previously would back down, and this quality has caused trouble for him at school. He continues with speech therapy and other therapy at home, but he is still able to deal with typical teenage situations. Like any precocious teenager, he has had his share of detentions at school, and if he is teased, he fights back. But he is dealing with his problems in a healthy way.

One day in the rehabilitation unit Brian told his mother, "I wish this was a bad dream and I could wake up." It is heartbreaking, but we all have to face the realities of life. Life is not fair, but we have the power to change things. I once heard a saying that now makes a great deal of sense in terms of head trauma, although it was originally mentioned in another context: "God doesn't give us what we want; He gives us what we need." We are not meant to understand the reasons. The challenge is face these problems and go on. Tragedy or adversity has brought families together and strengthened character when people are willing to accept it. I have seen so much courage and seemingly miraculous recoveries due to faith. I know that I was allowed to come back from death for a purpose, and my writing here is a part of that.

In considering Brian's recovery, much credit must be given to his therapists and nurses. When he arrived at the rehabilitation center, he was evaluated and immediately began physical, occupational, and speech therapy. The family was continually informed about his progress, and the atmosphere was always positive and encouraging. As he improved, he eventually returned home after seven months, and the therapy continued at home and in school. He is still improving, and there is no limit to how far he can go.

Brian's story is another piece in the puzzle of understanding head trauma. There are many differences between his experiences and those of others mentioned in this book. For example, there was no real memory loss (other than for a couple of weeks prior to and following the accident), and he seemed to be much the same child. However, there are many similarities that we all share. Treatment varies according to the specific needs of the patient, but the techniques can be used for all of us in similar ways. The major target is the brain, teaching it to function "normally." Cognitive training, directed at relearning the thought process, is invaluable for integration into society. The Brians among us will appreciate how lucky we are to have benefited from what medical science is learning and how bright our futures can be.

Jerry

Jerry, age 15, was hit by a van in June 1984 and dragged 30 feet, sustaining multiple injuries, with the onset of seizures and unconsciousness in addition to profuse bleeding around the face and damage to the right hand and forearm. He was taken to a trauma center hospital where he remained for one month before being transferred to a children's rehabilitation center for four months.

Jerry was walking in a parking lot when he was hit by a van and dragged many feet before being trapped under the van for at least 20 minutes. It was fortunate that he was taken immediately to the trauma center. He suffered from a lack of oxygen because he was not given oxygen in the ambulance. He responded only to deep pain stimulation. Surgery was performed immediately to save his right arm. The left side of his body was paralyzed as a result of the impact of the right side of his head with the van's windshield. Because of a hematoma, his vision would be impaired. The only undamaged parts of Jerry's body were one leg and his spine.

Jerry was taken to the same trauma center as Nancy (to be discussed) and Brian. Although he was in a coma for about one and one-half weeks, he did not "lighten up" gradually; he seemed to wake up immediately.

Once Jerry had emerged from the coma, the extent of the damage to his memory could be determined. He amazed everyone with details of past experiences, yet he readily forgot that he had had lunch five minutes before. Jerry's parents worked with him, helping him to carry out range of motion exercises, providing sneakers to prevent foot drop, and supplying batteries for his Walkman radio.

Like David's mother, Jerry's mother kept a diary of progress, an invaluable help in reconstructing what had happened. In reading both I found many pages that were virtually identical. It was as though I were rereading the account that David's mother had written.

For example, both mothers related that their sons did not like physical therapy (neither did I). They both fell asleep during these sessions. On the first day in physical therapy Jerry was taken from his wheelchair by two therapists, placed onto a tilt table, and strapped into place so that he could not thrash around. (The tilt table is used to adjust the patient to an upright position as a first step in maintaining balance and eventually walking.) As the table was tilted to an upright position, Jerry began screaming. Because he complained that he was dizzy and would vomit, the therapists lowered the table slightly.

Response:

A tilt table looks like a doctor's examining table which is able to move from horizontal to vertical. A patient is strapped in to keep him from slipping or falling forward as the table elevates. The table is used to gradually and safely elevate the patient who has been in bed or sitting for a prolonged period of time. This may take minutes or days. Vital signs (pulse, blood pressure, respiration) are carefully monitored by the therapist, since patients may experience nausea, dizziness, or vomiting (like Jerry) with the change of position.

—Maria Kendricken

Jerry's mother stayed with him while the therapist worked with several other patients. Jerry continued his shouting until he eventually tired and fell asleep. After a couple of sessions, however, he had mastered the tilt table and was ready for the parallel bars. Like

David, Jerry needed assistance because of his weakened side. He was supported, and the therapist would push his left leg forward with her foot after Jerry had moved his right foot forward. Even walking the short distance of the bars was enough to exhaust him, yet he was proud of what he had accomplished.

The occupational therapist used a series of standardized techniques that both David and I encountered. Jerry had to stack and unstack cones, put marbles or pegs into appropriate holes, and match designs of colored blocks. Although it was difficult for him, he was usually able to perform these activities after several tries.

Response:

The use of stacking cones, marbles and pegs, and matching block designs represents a tabletop or transfer of training treatment approach. Although this approach is sometimes effectively used today, generally occupational therapists use a more functional neurodevelopmental or sensory integrative approach to treating perceptual, coordination, cognitive, and other deficits. More detailed information on these treatment approaches appears later in the book. In addition, the reader is referred to the references for additional information.[1-5]

—Barbara Zoltan

These therapies, along with others, were used at the trauma center, starting only several days after Jerry's emergence from the coma. Even then the family noticed many differences in his behavior. For example, he had normally been a very quiet and introverted teenager, musical and artistic. His two brothers, one older and one younger, contrasted greatly by being very hyperactive and extremely vocal. Jerry had been the buffer between them. However, after the coma, all that changed. He became quite vocal.

Once, when his mother stood at his left side, supposedly his blind side, Jerry saw her. Of course his vision was blurred, but he did see her, and with his glasses on he could see her clearly. Thereafter Jerry always wanted to keep his glasses on, even when he fell asleep. When his mother tried to remove the glasses so that he would not break them in thrashing around in his sleep, Jerry immediately woke up and hollered for his glasses. It seems as though he just did not want to miss anything, evidence of his assertiveness and desire to know every detail of what was happening around him.

His ability to recognize people was unaffected, but his mother had to teach him how to tell time. Apparently the part of the brain that stores this information was damaged. He also had days and nights of confusion. The greatest problem was his short term memory. He would eat, and then eat again, unaware that he had just had a full meal. Thus his eating had to be controlled.

The intensive treatment began after Jerry was transferred to the rehabilitation center. He had been able to get around by learning to get into and out of a wheelchair. The physical therapy was outlined when he arrived: "The patient is to receive physical therapy for progressive ambulation training and more general hand range of motion and to insure full range of motion of all affected joints except for that which still has the pin in it." Other types of therapy were used as his abilities progressively increased.

Jerry's resistance to physical therapy is common in victims of head trauma. His dislike was evidenced by his conveniently forgetting how to find the therapy room. He would arrive late or miss the therapy session entirely. However, that soon changed. He tired of listening to the therapists' complaints. Even though they required him to work to the limit of his endurance, he liked them and wanted to please them. They had become his friends.

Speech therapy was more fun. During one session Jerry was sitting at a computer with the therapist by his side. He was typing a list of 10 random words that he had been studying, trying to remember the words in proper sequence and how to spell them correctly. The computer immediately let him know whether he was right or wrong, and the therapist repeatedly gave him verbal cues. When the lesson was fun, as with my training, the results were always positive. For any average teenager, playing computer or video games is very enjoyable, especially when one's level of skill mastery improves. Jerry was eager to repeat this feeling of satisfaction and wished to "play" often.

Some of Jerry's physical therapy sessions were enjoyable, at least to his family. He went through many of the same procedures that I encountered. For example, he had to try knocking the therapist off balance, and Jerry was just as successful as I had been. Although he was exhausted, he stayed awake. At times the therapy was actually painful, as he tried to stretch and move muscles that refused to move. Then it was discovered that he needed training sessions to eliminate double vision. Apparently the most productive therapy was visiting at home on weekends, therapy both for Jerry and for his family.

The accident happened in June 1984. On an unusually warm December day that year Jerry, at first unsteadily, peddled his bicycle on the boardwalk. He had been close to death, but now he was very much alive. Today he is a typical teenager. One would hardly guess what he has been through. There is still evidence of his accident, but with time and effort more of the deficiencies may disappear. As with so many victims of head trauma, the road to recovery is difficult. Recovery does not occur overnight. However, every case I have seen strengthens my conviction that determination, love, and persistence can work miracles.

Darren

Darren was hit by a car in May 1985. He was in a coma for one to two weeks, in an intensive care unit for one month, and in the hospital for less than two months. He was transferred to a pediatric rehabilitation center for one month and then went home on weekends. This was followed by daily outpatient therapy.

Darren was 15 when he was hit by a car while walking across the street. He was thrown onto another car, head first. He was taken to a hospital that unfortunately was not a registered trauma center, although it was advertised as such. Although there was very slight physical damage, he was in a deep coma for almost two weeks until he began to emerge. By the beginning of July, two months after the accident, he was able to be transferred to a rehabilitation facility. It is hard to believe, but, other than from his family, Darren received no physical therapy during his stay at the hospital.

During his coma Darren's family noted that although he responded to those around him, he seemed calmer when family members were with him. When he began to thrash around in bed, members of the family would speak to him gently and quiet him down so that he did not require Valium®. During this time the family was allowed to visit at any time, and they took full advantage of the opportunity. The nurses were pleased because the family did so much of the work. Doctors were reluctant to give any information, probably because they had no definitive answers. The information they did give was rather negative because no one knew what to expect. Family members had to rely on their faith and their family strength.

The physical damage was minimal; a small bone in one arm was broken and a shoulder was dislocated. However, while in the hospital Darren developed spinal meningitis and a urinary tract infection.

Darren was unable to communicate until after he left the hospital, and his memory at that time was severely impaired. He first began to improve when he was with his family and in fact walked on the beach nine days before the therapists told the family that he was walking. He spoke to his parents several days before the speech therapist reported the exciting news that Darren had spoken for the first time.

During the hospital stay nothing was done by the staff in regard to rehabilitation except for about 20 minutes of range of motion exercises. Members of the family were surprised to see that after a week in the hospital, Darren had not even been raised in bed. There were no therapists on the staff, although the hospital had been advertised as a trauma center. Because no effort had been made to feed him orally, his parents started feeding him ice cream. Finally he progressed enough so that the feeding tube could be removed. His mother did so much of the work that the nurses seemed to assume that it was her job, and they did little to help her. His mother served as a private duty nurse, bathing him, changing his sheets, and feeding him. A student nurse found a wheelchair when no one else could seem to find one, so at least he could be moved around.

At this time Darren had temporarily lost his sense of taste, and favorite foods did not interest him. He was like a baby, having to be fed. His therapy ended at four o'clock, with time wasted afterward as far as his parents were concerned. They of course were eager for him to come home so that they could work with him.

A few days after admission to the pediatric rehabilitation unit, therapy began. It was obvious that Darren was less than thrilled, for he bit the therapist. That particular therapist, it turned out, did not work well with Darren, not because she did not know her job but because she was so business-like and stern that she failed to gain Darren's cooperation. He displayed a great deal of hostility and lack of cooperation, but he worked well with other therapists, who joked and talked more kindly to him. It seemed that almost everyone on the staff carried out their jobs strictly "by the book," with no room for flexibility. The impression was that the therapist could do no wrong. Darren was treated like a seven year old without regard for his developmental or chronological age, mainly because that was the actual age of most of the other patients. Staff members were not equipped to deal with, nor were they familiar with, "children" of Darren's size or maturity. There were no neuropsychologists, and when Darren's mother asked about this, she was told that the social worker doubled as the neuropsychologist.

Eventually the family tired of fighting the system. After one month they began bringing Darren home every evening and working with him there. They geared their therapy sessions to his interests, and he worked hard for them. Because the family was close and knew Darren well, they instinctively knew how to do for him what the rehabilitation staff members were not doing. They set goals, such as having him walking by August, and he accomplished them.

Darren's memory loss was for the immediate past, and as in cases mentioned previously, he could not remember anything immediately after it happened. His father visted one day and left the room for a few minutes. When he returned, Darren greeted him as if he had not seen him since the previous day. To compensate for his memory loss, his parents brought a Polaroid camera and took many pictures, including visitors and meals, and put the photographs on the walls to remind Darren of what he had done each day. For example, they would take a picture of a visitor and write the date and time on the photograph so that Darren would know when the friend had been there. The family started a log for him so that he could later try to piece together what he had done. Using the pictures proved successful, if only to reassure Darren about what had happened and lessen his anxiety and frustration over not remembering. Perhaps this technique would be useful for others with short term memory loss.

In regard to walking, the family again took matters into their own hands. I have mentioned that with their help Darren was walking on the beach in the evening long before the therapist encouraged him to walk. His parents had set goals for him, and Darren strove to achieve them. He wanted to please them as well as feel a sense of accomplishment, most likely because they had done so much for him.

Response:

Although Darren may not have been walking in therapy, his physical therapist may have been working with him on activities that precede walking, such as balancing, alignment in standing posture, and taking a few steps. Attention is paid to the quality of walking to correct deviations that ultimately prevent bad habits. As a result, this should allow the patient to walk more normally. Families should check with the therapist who will teach them the best way to walk with the patient and carry over what has been emphasized in treatment.

—Maria Kendricken

Soon his family set another goal, this one seemingly impossible to achieve — that Darren would be back in school right after Christmas vacation. Instead he returned right after Thanksgiving vacation, a month earlier. His short term memory improved rapidly with the concentrated help of his family. He was ready.

In less than eight months Darren was back in the 4H Club, even going on weekend trips. The only real problem was that he tired easily, a common effect of head trauma. It is almost impossible now to single him out as being different from his peers, thanks to the love and guidance of those closest to him.

Darren's experiences raise several questions useful in treating all victims of head trauma: How do families protect themselves from incompetent care? How can they be assured that the staff is doing its job and not leaving its responsibilities to others? How can a family be sure that the hospital and rehabilitation care unit are best suited for their needs?

Unfortunately Darren cannot now benefit from what his family learned from their experiences, but future victims of head trauma will. Although it may take some effort on the part of the family involved in such a case, they must find out exactly what resources are available. For example, an accident victim obviously will be taken first to the nearest hospital, but when there is a choice, it should be a registered trauma center. If there is time to choose a rehabilitation center, it is not difficult to find out how many therapists, neuropsychologists, and nurses are on the staff and the techniques of rehabilitation they use. A little research can save much aggravation later.

Another point Darren's family proved was the power of positive thinking. In the beginning they were told not to think about the idea of Darren's walking for at least nine months. They would not accept this and they proved everyone wrong. However, one must remember that all families are not like Darren's. What happens with other families or patients without families? Darren's family's experiences only confirm the need for information. Hospitals should supply resource material and directions for help to those concerned. Sorry to say, although my name and telephone number are listed with every trauma center in my area, I have rarely been called. The "why" is not important. What is important is that this situation be corrected.

Nancy

Nancy, age 17, was a passenger in a car hit by a truck in October 1985. Her car in turn collided with another car, and she was trapped inside the car for a half hour. Nancy was in a coma for about two weeks; she stayed in the hospital for five weeks and then was transferred to a rehabilitation center.

Nancy was on her way to school when the car in which she was riding was hit by a truck and pushed into another car. She was in shock and was trapped in the car until she was removed by the "Jaws of Life" and received excellent care by the paramedics. Their competent treatment included establishing an airway, starting an intravenous infusion, and assisting her breathing with a respiration bag. Time is an important factor in trauma, yet Nancy had been in shock for more than 30 minutes! She was in a coma and had internal bleeding, but she appeared to be all right otherwise. At that time the doctors and nurses thought that she would be in a coma for only a couple of days. After a few days, however, Nancy's mother learned the cold hard facts. Because of the length of time Nancy had been in shock, staff members were worried. Her eyes opened in less than one week, but she did not begin to emerge from the coma until after about two weeks. Prior to this the neurosurgeon gave her about a 10 percent chance of waking up at all. As in David's case, there is the ethical question of what a doctor should or should not tell the family of a patient. Is it best to try to predict accurately what will happen? The family must realize that the doctor's opinion is not necessarily the final word.

Response:

It is difficult for doctors to predict recovery. Many have tried and been proven wrong. Neurologists and physicians use standardized specific evaluations such as the Glasgow Coma Scale. This scale helps to determine prognosis, but every patient progresses at their own pace and may plateau for a while. Recovery will usually still occur many years after injury.

—Maria Kendricken

Nancy's mother is a nurse, but she was not familiar with the problems posed by trauma. Her nursing background may have been an asset, but she admits that strong faith and tenacity kept her going. During the five weeks in the hospital Nancy practiced range of motion exercises with the aid of her therapists and her family, but as in my case, there was resistance. Nancy was fortunate, as I had been, to have sustained no serious bodily damage. She also had the advantage of a private duty nurse around the clock in the beginning.

One of the nurses, in particular, was exceptional, for she was familiar with head trauma cases and worked hard in helping Nancy, in addition to being a "patient advocate" in regard to treatment and care. The average patient is not aware of his rights and the facilities offered in a hospital. For example, such a simple matter as long term parking is almost never discussed. The family also has to be informed about such matters as social workers and counseling help.

Anyone hospitalized for any length of time is faced with common problems, which can be overcome early if the staff and family are alert. For example, pressure sores, foot drop, and arm contractures, often a result of such confinement, can be avoided with proper care. However, these problems are often overlooked because the staff is too busy with life-and-death situations and families do not know what to look for.

In the beginning, after the coma, Nancy could not even hold up her head. She could not speak then, but she learned to write things down. This was a tiresome procedure, but it worked. Everything exhausted her quite readily, another common feature in head trauma, and thus learning took place slowly at first. She does not remember clearly the period when she was in the hospital or what was done during her therapy sessions, but her mother was there constantly, having moved into the rehabilitation center when Nancy was transferred there. Her mother had thoroughly investigated every rehabilitation center in the area, never hesitating to ask questions or make requests.

In learning what happened to her, I gained many ideas to pass along to other families. Because Nancy's mother was a nurse, she was not intimidated by doctors and other professional people and was not afraid to question their judgments. She was also blessed with a strong faith and opinions about what was best for her daughter. In addition she learned that insurance is a vital factor in treatment. It is sad to say, but "money talks." Everyone should try to obtain the best insurance available as a precaution. No one knows when tragedy can strike, and it is often too late when we hear, "Why didn't I get insurance?"

Nancy's mother has no reservations about speaking out. She came up with many other helpful suggestions. First, the patient should be allowed to go home on weekends. In every case I have known of this has been a factor that has speeded recovery and helped the family to come to terms with the problem. Second visitors should not be restricted.

Response:
In general, family and friends should be allowed to visit and participate in treatment. In some cases, however, progress can be hampered if the patient is angry at a family member or too distracted by family to participate in the program. Some visitors will try to sneaking in alcohol or drugs which are physically harmful to the patient (especially after head trauma), and these must be restricted.

—Maria Kendricken

Although doctors and therapists may frown on this idea, visitors are an important part of therapy. Too often friends forget the patient after a long period has passed. They must be encouraged to help the patient adjust. Third, learn to deal with fear. Counseling is invaluable for the patient and the family. Most important, check to see what kinds of help are available. There are many therapeutic and counseling programs, and financial help is to be found if one does some research.

The rest of Nancy's story is no less than miraculous. In less than five months she returned to high school on a part-time basis and expects to graduate with her class. She continues to report for therapy every day and sees a counselor three times a week. She is still improving, and the therapy has not slowed her life down. Nancy was invited to five proms and is enjoying life to the fullest. She came out of the tragedy with no memory loss (other than for the brief period during and following the accident), and she is as bright and bubbly as ever. She is one of the rare victims of head trauma who come out of this ordeal well. She heard the doctor's "10 percent" prediction but refused to give up. Her future now is bright. Nancy wants to be a photographer after graduation, and no doubt she will reach that goal.

In reading this chapter you will have recognized examples from all points on the recovery scale. Although Nancy is near the top of the scale, others unfortunately will most likely remain near the bottom.

Ken

In May 1985 Ken was walking on steelwork (performing his job as an ironworker) when the girder inexplicably toppled, dropping him to the pavement on his head. He was in a coma for six weeks, and required a tracheostomy to breathe and a gastrostomy to receive food. When he emerged from the coma, he could not remember what had happened, nor recognize his girlfriend. It was several weeks before he could even begin to speak.

Within three months Ken was able to talk well, particularly about the rehabilitation program he was in. His memory returned, and though he was still often confused, his enthusiasm and desire to improve never wavered. Unlike many victims, he looked forward to physical therapy as well as occupational, recreational, and speech therapy, rehabilitation nursing, and psychological counseling. He delighted his therapists with his positive attitude and desire to cooperate.

Ken continued in the rehabilitation center until November, when he was released to return home under his girlfriend's care. However, he still returned to the center several times a week for further therapy.

It is now more than a year later. Ken can walk by himself, but still has trouble with balance. He is alert and oriented, can initiate some tasks, and seems to realize that what he is doing will help him overcome his deficits. This realization seems to have been a big plus for Ken. Because he understands why he is going through these therapy activities, he is willing to work hard to achieve success. Unfortunately, this level of insight is not common among victims of head trauma.

While Ken was in the rehabilitation facility he faced many frustrations. Knowing that he needed therapy was not enough to get the job done. In Ken's case, sometimes he could accomplish a task and other times he could not. He enjoyed being taught, but somehow his brain would become "short-circuited" and he would be unable to do what he wanted to do.

Often Ken would talk in a series of non sequiturs, making an appropriate remark and then wandering to totally unrelated points. Fortunately, he is aware of this problem and works to stay on the subject.

According to his girlfriend, Ken's attitudes and actions are totally different from those she used to know. Typical of his job, he had been rugged and very macho. He fought for his ideas and would not accept any interference from anyone. Today he is easygoing and gentle. This is uncommon among head injured patients, who often become more aggressive and demanding. All those who know Ken say that he now talks differently, walks differently, and acts differently. The differences are not subtle; there has been a total personality change.

Ken was very athletic before his accident, a tough and aggressive competitor. Today he channels his energies into a sport learned during recreational therapy — swimming. His only competitor is himself. Swimming has taught him to overcome many physical and cognitive difficulties. He has shown reduced spasticity, improved relaxation, greater mobility and independence, improved head control, and increased breathing control. More important, his self-esteem has improved because of his sense of accomplishment.

Today Ken continues to build his independence with the help of his girlfriend and the rehabilitation team that has been treating him. I learned a lot from Ken, and his story corroborates the opinions of others that determination is the key to rehabilitation. Although Ken will never go back to his job as an ironworker, he has the potential to lead a happy and fulfilling life. He is blessed with the ability to understand and accept his deficits, and has the love of someone who encourgaes him to try.

Much of Ken's story is unique among head trauma patients, but other aspects are typical. His refusal to accept the restaints of his disability can be an inspiration for others. His prognosis had been negative when he arrived at the hospital after his fall. Thank goodness Ken would not accept that!

Mary

Mary was in an automobile accident in March 1982 and was in a coma for three months. She sustained multiple physical injuries and brain damage, with short term memory loss. She was later transferred to a rehabilitation center where she remained for one year. After discharge she continued to receive outpatient therapy.

Mary was 16½ years old when she was practice-driving with her father near her home. An automobile collision occurred in which her head hit the side window and the steering wheel, although she was wearing her seat belt. Both Mary and her father were critically injured. They were taken to different hospitals because, they were told, they could receive better treatment if separated (the accident happened on a busy Saturday when hospitals are often understaffed). Because of her head injury, Mary was taken to the closest hospital. She required surgery for a hematoma, a tracheotomy to breathe, and surgical repair for multiple fractures and internal bleeding. She was not expected to live.

Her father was also in critical condition, but there was no head injury. After a lengthy stay at the hospital and six months of bed rest at home, he was able to resume his normal life. Mary, however, remained in a coma for three months and was fed by tube throughout this period. During this time her mother insisted on being with her as much as possible, although the hospital staff did not approve at first. After six to seven weeks Mary was transferred from the intensive care unit to the rehabilitation section of the hospital. Here her mother spent 17 to 18 hours a day with her.

Response:

As the author has previously stressed, family involvement is crucial for patient progress. The involvement, however, should be structured and balanced to benefit both the patient and the family. Mary's mother spending 17 or 18 hours a day with Mary is emotionallly and physically exhausting, and therefore is not healthy for Mary's mother. In time, family exhaustion turns into resentment and anger toward the patient, making the time the patient and family spend together no longer therapeutic.

—Barbara Zoltan

Although the medical care was excellent, the nurses were uncooperative. They repeatedly left Mary in wet diapers and soaking in perspiration for hours when her mother was not there. She thus took it upon herself to become Mary's private duty nurse. Mary was totally paralyzed, yet her mother received no help from the nursing staff in the simplest task of helping to turn her daughter to prevent pressure sores. Therapy and primary nursing care became less effective. No effort was made to prevent problems such as pressure sores, atrophy, or foot drop, which may have been avoidable.

The first sign of emergence from the coma came after three months when Mary's mother leaned down to kiss her, and Mary responded with a return kiss. She mouthed the words "Hi, Mom!" although she was unable to see. She started speaking, very softly and very quickly. Strangely enough, although she was born in the United States, she spoke in the language of her immigrant parents and thus no one on the staff could understand her. When her mother told her to speak in English, Mary responded, "They can learn how to speak this!"

The next four years involved a slow rehabilitation process. The extensive physical damage had to be dealt with first. Because private duty nurses were not allowed in the rehabilitation section of the hospital, Mary's mother did all the work herself. Mary had difficulty in learning new skills because her short term memory was severely impaired.

Even now her reactions and emotional responses are scrambled and inconsistent; some behavior is childlike, and some is mature.

Physical therapy took the most time because her paralyzed limbs resisted movement. Moreover, in the beginning she was not approached as the child she actually was. However, Mary understood the necessity for therapy and made the best of the situation. Not until recently have more advanced techniques been used in her treatment.

The therapy sessions throughout Mary's rehabilitation had one major drawback: The number of patients attending each session was too large, and thus there was little time for individual attention by the therapist. As a result Mary was "lost in the crowd." When she was instructed to perform a particular task and left alone, she often did not know what to do. This both frustrated and embarrassed her.

Mary's mother made an important discovery during this time: When a visitor arrives, one should not say to the patient, "Look who's here." This adds to the patient's frustration. Instead say, for example, "Look, Sally's here." In this way the patient does not have to be embarrassed when meeting someone he does not remember.

Occupational therapy and speech therapy, although enjoyable, were also frustrating for Mary. Constant supervision was necessary. Direct eye contact, pointing, and verbal cues were useful, but as soon as the therapist went to another patient, all was forgotten. Speech therapy was required to get Mary to speak louder and more slowly. She had to be reminded repeatedly to speak up and not garble her words.

Today Mary is living at home. Her physical problems are still evident. She has a brace on one leg, and one side is still paralyzed. She also still speaks very quietly and quickly. Her mind seems fragmented: At times she is very mature and intellectual, but the next minute she acts like a small child. She may answer a complex question appropriate to her age level and then be unable to understand a simple question that an ordinary toddler could answer. To provide help, Mary will be joining a health spa. Not only will she get needed therapy but also it will be more like fun than work for her.

Response:
Although Mary's joining a health spa has many social and emotional benefits which should be encouraged, the physical activities provided can be detrimental if unsupervised or provided without guidelines from a physical or occupational therapist. For example, resistive exercises and use of weights will increase abnormal tone and decrease function. It is heartbreaking for the family, patient, and therapist to see a patient attain a physical and functional level after months of rehabilitation only to lose this level after a few weeks of inappropriate physical activity.

—Barbara Zoltan

The toll this ordeal has taken on Mary's family is immense. Both parents work with her continually, day and night. Her mother hopes that someday Mary will be well again.

Her father, however, is more realistic. The most difficult problem is in dealing with the past. Pictures throughout the house and conversations with family members signify that the past has not been laid to rest.

Mary's case is all too common. Family members recall their past lives with fondness and find it difficult to accept the present or the future. All they can do is to cope. Family relationships are strained, and even getting up to face a new day is often tedious. A once promising future is shattered in an instant, and one's faith is put to the test.

Mary's future is uncertain because of her short term memory loss. She forgets almost immediately what has just been said, and thus continual repetition is necessary. However, there is hope, perhaps not that she will be able to do everything she once did but that she can progress to a higher level of independence so that she can manage with less need for constant watchful care. Mary is a loving girl who has much to offer. New techniques and programs being developed may help her to make progress and to become less of a burden to her family.

Nick

I saved the last case study until the end for a specific reason, for it exemplifies both ends of the spectrum. In dealing with head trauma, emotions run from total despair to jubilant hope. We must face the fact that some victims will never be able to function on their own, and will always need 24 hour care. The following case study is not about one specific person; it is a composite of the stories of several victims with similar disabilities.

Nick is in his midtwenties. Several years ago as a pedestrian he was struck by a speeding car, tossed over 30 feet and left for dead. Nick's skull was fractured and several limbs were broken. He remained in a coma for close to a year. He was in a rehabilitation center for a couple of years, but nothing further could be done for him there. He is presently in a nursing home, with the elderly and the senile, requiring around-the-clock care. He attends a rehabilitation program several days a week for therapy.

Relating Nick's story is difficult for me. The healthy, loving, caring man he was has been replaced by a prisoner trapped in the shell of a body. He cannot speak. He has learned sign language, and it is obvious that he can think and feel and care. However, his physical limitations are so profound that it is a slow and painful process for him just to sign a single word.

At first I was not going to include Nick's story in this chapter. But I realized that I cannot forget what can happen in dealing with head trauma. I had to put my personal feelings aside and describe what can happen, no matter how hopeless or depressing it may be. Nick's experiences have left his family in a continuing state of anxiety. They cannot help but remember what a good son he was, what a devoted, caring, vital person he had been. The heartbreak comes when one realizes that the same person, with all his outstanding qualities, is still inside that misshapen body, that he cannot speak and is tormented with seizures and long spells of sleep. He is fed through a tube. He can laugh at a joke and cry from frustration.

In dealing with all the Nicks in the world, we are faced with thoughts that we do not want to think. "He should have died in the accident rather than live like this. What did I do wrong that he should suffer this way? Maybe a miracle will happen." It cannot be determined who is suffering the most. Nick understands his condition but cannot control his fate. His family and friends love him, but they cannot give up; they are all trying to cope because they will never accept what has happened.

There is no answer. The only help can come from counseling and group support. Fortunately the Nicks are a minority. Many victims of head trauma go on to lead happy and productive lives. Some are blessed with the ability to return to their former lives with little difficulty.

Conclusion

The cases presented in this chapter vary in severity, but they share much in common. Each gives evidence of the need for more understanding of the victims of head trauma, particularly in terms of counseling for the family. Unresolved emotional problems can be detrimental to progress and must be faced. Mary's family is presently benefiting from counseling to resolve conflicts that have resulted from the accident.

If the patient is able to understand what is going on around him, he will also need such counseling to deal with frustration, depression, and guilt. Families in turn must learn not only to cope but to accept. Perhaps they can come to realize that they must let go and allow the patient the freedom to grow and develop to his maximal potential. Difficulties cannot be simplified; they can, however, be considered one by one and dealt with intelligently and objectively.

Response:

The head trauma patient should be placed on a structured head trauma unit where the environment is self-contained and in which a specially trained team of nurses, therapists, and physicians interact with the head trauma patients. Appendix B shows a list of questions that families should ask when choosing a head injury rehabilitation facility.

In his room each patient has a calendar with the days of the month crossed off, a clock, and a schedule board which they are encouraged to follow by themselves if able. If the patient is using a wheelchair, a schedule should be put on the armrest. There should be a reality board at the nurse's station with day and date, enabling the patients sitting at the nurse's station to see it. Familiar objects are brought from home into the patient's room (stuffed animals, posters, musical tapes, photographs) which put the patient at ease and may stimulate memory. Visitors are required to sign in and out on a dated sheet of paper posted in the patient's room, since the patient often may not recall having had visitors.

In therapy each patient should be seen on a one-on-one basis with the same therapists at the same times in the same small, quiet, softly lit room. This facilitates a carry-over of memory, less distractibility, consistency in responding to behaviors, and building up of trust, and enables the patient to lessen anxiety and participate more actively. In this environment therapeutic measures work on specfic physical deficits, memory problems, and distractibility. Therapy carries over from one discipline to the next. Patients are sometimes co-treated by two disciplines. Treatment begins slowly with structure and simple movements and tasks. A patient is always supervised and guided through a task until it is determined that he is independent enough to do the task. When able, the patient should be dressed for therapy. (Patients who have frequent bouts of bowel or bladder problems may be dressed in hospital gowns initially for ease in changing.) Once a patient beomes more independent and his memory improves, he may be placed in a group exercise or discussion situation which also helps socialization skills and provides support. Each patient is given a logbook in which entries are made by the patient (if able), family, and therapists. The logbook is a diary used to record the day's events and prompt the patient's memory.

Time spent in therapies is governed by the patient's level of physical endurance, attention, and agitation. The patient's tolerance for therapy sessions may be very brief at first, perhaps only 10 minutes at a time. The patient can be seen several times daily for short periods; eventually the number of sessions is gradually decreased.

Patients are given breaks during longer treatment sessions. Therapies in an intensive program often begin early in the morning for bathing and dressing, and usually end late in the afternoon. After dinner time is given for recreation, relaxation, and family support. There are recreational activities such as video games, cards, television, and musical entertainment. Families who visit in the evenings are encouraged to review the day's events (such as showering and feeding) and to walk with the patient when he is ready.

Families should be involved in the rehabilitation program from the very beginning. Families are encouraged to attend therapy sessions and to participate by actually getting the patient dressed and undressed and into and out of the bed, car, and toilet. A family conference where all team members report to the family is scheduled during the first week after admission.

Families should attend family education classes in the evenings (if available). These classes teach the family about head trauma, the team approach, and specific involvement of each discipline. The team members also answer questions and provide support.

Patients are encouraged to get out of the hospital on weekends, and are given day passes (if medically stable). The family may take the patient out for a car ride, to a restaurant, or home to practice learned activities.

In most cases visits are made to the patient's home to assess the patient's functional skills in his own environment, make recommendations for purchasing equipment or changing the environment, and help determine how independently a patient can function.

Separate out-trips should be made available as part of the rehabilitation program. One these trips therapists take patients (either individually or in a group) into the community to practice activities and strategies, such as walking in crowds and using money and socialization skills.

Prior to being discharged the patient may be placed on a phase-out program on the nursing unit. This allows the patient and the primary caretaker to practice functional skills which are necessary for discharge (i.e., simulating the home environment by making the patient responsible for dressing, showering, making the bed, asking for medications on time, etc.).

Some programs include a therapeutic overnight visit which allows the patient to spend one night away from the hospital while remaining an inpatient. The patient goes home overnight with the family to practice functional skills and returns to the hospital the following day. During the patient's remaining days in the hospital the therapists can work with the patient and family on any problems that have arisen.

Therapy usually continues after the patient is discharged to the home. The patient may receive therapy in the home through an agency such as the Visiting Nurse's Association or a more extensive outpatient community reentry program that specifically meets the needs of the head trauma population. The program's activities are geared toward helping the patient make the transition from the hospital to the community.

Depending on the patient's needs, therapy may be provided on a one-on-one basis to continue the progress made as an inpatient. In addition, therapies focus on group activities as a means of attaining the required skills to be independent in the home or work place. Groups facilitate appropriate socialization skills and provide peer support. They incorporate several cognitive tasks at once. Groups that are currently being offered at some facilities include:

1) Therapeutic work program: Patients are supervised in a work-type environment. They may type, make copies, file, deliver mail, and update bulletin boards.

2) Community out-trips: Patients are taught to use public transportation, follow a map, shop for food or clothes, and appreciate cultural experiences.

3) Newspaper groups: Patients work as reporters, journalists, and editors of a newspaper circulated in the hospital.

4) Patient-family nights: A family member pairs up with a patient from another family. The group may go to a mall or restaurant or out for evening entertainment. The experience enables both the patient and family to learn and gain support from one another.

5) Coordination groups: Patients focus on skills needed for functional mobility and leisure activities, such as swimming, running, and dancing.

Vocational counseling is continued in outpatient status to aid the patient's return to school or workplace. A driving program may be available. The program usually consists of a written and practical exam with recommendations and follow-up treatment given as needed.

Outpatient therapy may last weeks, months, or years, depending on a patient's needs.

—Maria Kendricken

References

1. Zoltan B, Siev E, Freisthat B: Perceptual and Cognitive Dysfunction of the Adult Stroke Patient. Thorofare, NJ, Slack, Incorporated, 1986.

2. Ayres AJ: Sensory Integration and Learning Disorders. Los Angeles, CA, Western Psychological Services, 1980.

3. Bobath B: Adult Hemiplegia: Evaluation and Treatment. Ed 2. London, William Heinemann Medical Books, 1978.

4. Davies PM: Steps to Follow. Berlin, Springer Verlag, 1985.

5. Carr J, Shepherd R: Motor Relearning Programme for Stroke. Rockville, MD, Aspen Publications, 1983.

4

Speaking Out
The Families' Survey

The case studies in this book have yielded many suggestions for improvement of the treatment presently offered to victims of head trauma and their families. In this chapter I will discuss some of the problems resulting from lack of knowledge and misunderstanding and their possible remedies.

My goal is to combat ignorance. We who have sustained head trauma arc the victims, and it is time for us to be heard. No one else can know what we are going through. Flexibility is the true sign of progress, and thus if traditional techniques have not been successful in promoting rapid recovery or rehabilitation back into society, other methods must be tried.

Many dedicated professionals understand what is happening and work hard to help, but by themselves individuals cannot change the overall system, with its instances of nursing "burn-out," overloaded schedules, and unacceptable nurse-patient ratios. These are but a few of the problems facing us.

The case studies show that the family plays a vital role in rehabilitation, but unfortunate victims who have no family or whose family will not participate need a program of treatment too. There is also the harsh but undeniable fact that many victims cannot obtain good treatment without insurance and a high income. What happens to the family when the wage earner is injured? Is help available for the patient and the family members when the time comes to live again with someone who has become a totally different person? Too little attention has been given to the family members who have to deal with the victim of head trauma.

Other pressing questions arise. How does one choose the best facility for the patient's needs? Indeed, what questions should be asked? How can a relative help in the patient's recovery? Is the setting of goals a useful technique, or does this merely lead to frustration?

To answer questions like these I devised the questionnaire shown in Appendix E to elicit information from relatives of victims of head trauma. A total of 150 people were sent these questionnaires, and 100 responded. The qualification for inclusion in this informal study was that the respondent had to be closely related to a head trauma victim — a parent, child, or spouse. The questionnaires were presented at head trauma support group meetings and seminars as well as to individuals.

Even before I distributed the questionnaires it was obvious that the families had an overwhelming desire to talk. Everyone was excited that people were actually interested in listening to their stories. Patients were also eager to talk (see Chapter 5). All family members seemed to share a common outlook, searching for answers. The following discussions summarize the findings in the survey.

Survey Results

The Sources of Information (Question 1)

1. What is your relationship to the patient?

The majority of answers came from a parent or the patient's spouse. This is logical since most of the patients were under age 34.

Accident Demographics (Questions 2, 3, 4)

2. What caused the head trauma?
3. In what year did the accident occur?
4. When you received news of the accident, did you know whom to call for information?

The survey revealed, not surprisingly, that motor vehicle accidents are the most common cause of head trauma — automobile collisions with pedestrians, bicycle and motorcycle riders, as well as with other automobiles. One accident resulted from a fight, and in another case a stroke occurred during brain surgery. One accident occurred as long ago as 1979, but the majority occurred in 1984 and 1985.

In most cases the relatives of the patient did not know where to turn for information on receiving news of the accident. Most families felt panic, helpless, and lost in not knowing what had happened or where to go for help. Although in most cases they eventually were able to function rationally, help was needed at the very beginning.

Residual Effects of Trauma (Questions 28, 29, and 32)

28. Did the patient suffer long term or short term memory loss?
29. Was there a personality change in the patient? If "yes," please describe briefly.
32. Was there a great deal of physical damage other than the head trauma?

In regard to memory loss, many patients forgot large blocks of time but did not have total amnesia as I did. The majority forgot the events surrounding the accident and had short term memory loss. Events in the distant past became more vivid, whereas the morning meal might be forgotten immediately.

It was difficult to determine whether physical limitations had an effect on the mental progress of the patient. However, in most cases the patient underwent a change in personality. Lack of inhibition, anger, frustration, and aggression were common, and these aspects were most difficult for family members to accept. In many cases they discovered that they were living with a new person, often one who was not very nice.

Dealing with these changes takes love, understanding, and professional help. Webster's dictionary defines trauma as "an emotional shock that creates substantial and lasting damage to the psychological development of the individual something that severely jars the mind or emotions." Such a shock rarely leaves the patient unscarred emotionally, and these scars exist as well in those closest to the patient. Years of living with a calm, easy-going child, for example, make life with an impulsive, disruptive, obnoxious child almost unbearable.

Hospital Facilities and Policies (Questions 6, 8)

6. Was long term parking made available for you and your relatives at the hospital?
8. Were you allowed liberal or unlimited visiting privileges?

In most cases long term parking was not made available for the patient's relatives at the hospital. When one considers that most of the patients were hospitalized for at least one or two months, parking costs could be enormous. After one mother had paid $6 a day for parking for more than a month, she found out unexpectedly from a guard that the hospital provided all-day parking for $1 for relatives of long term patients. Frequently, even when parking was available, the information was not volunteered. There is a great need for help in the hospital from the start in anticipating such questions that one normally would not even think of asking.

Visiting privileges in most cases were liberal or unlimited. However, several hospitals were very strict, particularly in regard to patients in intensive case units where in one instance only one relative was allowed to visit for five minutes each hour. In that case, when the family questioned the policy and made demands, the restrictions were often lifted. According to the survey, others silently complied, although they were unhappy about it. All too often families were intimidated by authority and did not make their feelings known.

Family Relationships with the Hospital Staff (Questions 7, 10, 11, 12, 14)

7. Was someone immediately available for you and your relatives to speak with when you arrived at the hospital?

10. Were you told precisely what to expect in regard to medical procedures?

11. Was the topic of "brain damage" discussed or even thought of in the beginning?

12. Were the doctors and nurses positive, negative, or noncommittal about recovery?

14. Were you told about the specific procedures to be used by each therapist and doctor?

Through conversations with those responding to the survey I learned that some were told the details of the accident and what was being done in response, but many questions were not answered. Some relatives came to the hospital only to wait and worry. The information obtained depended in part on the size of the hospital, its location, and the quality of its staff.

In regard to specific therapeutic procedures — range of motion exercises, the use of tilt tables and parallel bars, hand-eye coordination, and cognitive retraining — some doctors and therapists had neither the time nor the inclination to discuss such matters, and answers usually were given in technical terms that only another physician could understand. By contrast, some families were kept well informed. Others had to be aggressive in getting information. Still others, who did not persist, were told little or nothing. Once the critical period was over, family members received more information. However, it is during the crucial period immediately following the accident that questions like these should have been answered. Unfortunately the layman cannot possibly think of all the questions to ask at such a time, and the answers were not volunteered in many of these cases. Many dedicated doctors and nurses, however, do take the time to explain medical treatment to families of victims of head trauma.

The subject of brain damage is almost always thought of, but perhaps the question of damage to the head is not raised immediately because relatives are too much in shock to imagine the possibility of such an injury. Even the term concussion fails to raise the possibility of brain damage in many minds. For many people the term does not convey a sense of danger. The terms skull fracture and brain hemorrhage seem to carry more serious implications. However, such terms as head trauma or head injury are finally attracting attention.

Patients' relatives reported that doctors tended to be negative in their comments about the prognosis for recovery, whereas nurses tended to be more positive. Although it is relatively easy to predict whether the patient is going to live, the quality of his future life is often unknown. Probably the best approach for the physician is to be straightforward, to explain the situation in terms the family can understand and discuss the possible outcomes, admitting to not knowing the final answers. Thus the doctor or nurse makes the family aware of the range of possibilities — both best and worst outcomes — without being more specific. In turn family members must face reality but should not give up hope.

Therapy (Questions 9, 15, 34)

9. Was physical therapy given during coma? If "yes," what was done?

15. Was the patient examined by a psychologist or psychiatrist?

34. Aside from physical limitations, what was the greatest problem to overcome?

It used to be believed that the patient in coma is unaware of what is going on around him. Now it is known that the patient is indeed aware, and today family members and other visitors are encouraged to speak to the patient, play his favorite music, and so on. Progressive hospitals now also begin therapy during coma. Range of motion exercises are done throughout the coma period to keep the joints in motion and prevent muscle atrophy.

In most of the cases reported in my survey the patient was not examined by a psychiatrist or psychologist during the hospital stay. Once the patient was transferred to a rehabilitation center, he was examined and evaluated, but frequently the results of the evaluation were put aside and not referred to again. In the newer facilities a greater effort has been made recently to correct this problem.

Psychological problems were often mentioned as major issues as were memory loss and social adjustment. The answers on the survey revealed a widespread need for counseling for the patient and his family.

The Role of the Staff (Questions 19, 20, 22, 23, 26, and 27)

19. Was there a team effort among the therapists, or did each work independently? Was the family involved?

20. Was the nursing care adequate?

22. Were the daily routines performed by primary nurses or by licensed practical nurses?

23. Was the primary nurse aware of the patient's progress, or was her case load too great for her to give close attention?

26. Was any effort made to determine the mental age of the patient?

27. If "yes," was the patient treated like a child of that age?

Although most responses acknowledged a team effort on the part of the therapists, the family was not usually included. Each therapist seemed to be aware of the patient's progress in other therapy programs, however. The patient often responded better to one therapist than to others, and progress was achieved accordingly. Because of the patients' often childlike behavior, they would throw tantrums, avoid therapy sessions whenever possible, or be totally unreceptive if there was a personality conflict with the therapist. By contrast, the patient often progressed far beyond expectations with a therapist he liked and wanted to please.

The adequacy of nursing care varied with the hospital. As in all professions, there are both good and bad aspects. In one facility nurses watched television soap operas in a back room while patients screamed for attention. One child was left unattended, strapped to a toilet, while the nurse was smoking and chatting with others. In other hospitals nurses went out of their way to help, give consolation to families, and speak to administrators about the rights of the patients and their families. All too often, however, family members or private duty nurses took over many of the hospital nurses' responsibilities. Not uncommonly relatives, particularly the mother, carried out daily routines with the patient. In other cases a licensed practical nurse did the work, particularly in large understaffed hospitals.

In almost all cases the primary nurses seemed to be aware of the patient's progress, even though their case loads were often too large. Although there were isolated incidents in which the patient was ignored, this was rare, especially with a patient who was hospitalized for a considerable length of time. Patients who were hospitalized for a month or more soon developed rapport with the nurses.

Usually an effort was made to determine the patient's learning development level, particularly in recent cases. However, the patient was still treated and spoken to as one might a person of that chronological age. I was 48 at the time of my accident, yet I had the learning development level of an infant. When people talked to me, however, they spoke to the "old me," often only speaking more slowly or more loudly. Someone who is unfamiliar with head trauma sees an adult and expects to talk with an adult.

In all but a few cases the patient was not treated like a child of the appropriate learning development level. Therapists sometimes did not recognize the rapid change in their patients' learning development levels and continued to treat them as young children. Such patients often had the impression that they were being talked down to or patronized. In recent years progressive rehabilitation units have begun to watch for evidence of this developmental change and treat patients accordingly.

The Family's Role (Questions 5, 18, 35, 36, 37, 38, and 43)

5. Did you have any say in the emergency treatment of the patient?

18. Were you encouraged to help in the therapy (e.g., occupational therapy, physical therapy)?

35. Did you participate in any of the therapy sessions with the patient?

36. Did you work with the patient after therapy time (evenings and weekends)?

37. Did you have to work with the patient on your own, or were you encouraged by the therapists to do so?

38. Was the patient allowed home on weekends from rehabilitation? If "yes," did the patient and the family react in a positive way? Did the patient want to go back to the hospital after these visits?

43. What was the single greatest adjustment the family had to make in response to the patient's head trauma?

Most families were not consulted in regard to emergency treatment. They signed the release forms, but treatment was undertaken at the discretion of the physicians. Most relatives were intimidated and did not challenge the doctors' decisions. However, several — specifically in health related fields — did speak up and had a say in regard to what was done.

During occupational and physical therapy sessions most relatives were discouraged from participating but were encouraged to work with the patient on weekends or in the evenings. Almost half in my survey were told to leave the therapy to the therapists, who knew what they were doing. Nonetheless, family members who insisted on playing a role in therapy often were allowed to do so. Even when this was not encouraged by the staff, most relatives, particularly parents, wanted to help with therapy.

When physically capable, almost all the patients were permitted to go home on weekend visits, and usually this had beneficial effects. Frequently the patient did not want to go back to the hospital, but it was usually necessary. Many family members remembered that the usual complaint from the patient in the hospital was "I want to go home."

Whether dealing with a totally different personality, the limitations imposed on the patient, or a new life style, the greatest adjustment the family had to make was acceptance. Many families cannot accomodate these changes, but those in our sample were trying or had succeeded. However, they represent only a small percentage of those involved with victims of head trauma.

Counseling and Ancillary Programs (Questions 13, 16, 17, 24, 25, and 33)

13. Was someone available to discuss insurance and legal matters with you and your family?

16. Was counseling available for the patient?

17. Was counseling available for the family?

24. If the patient was the breadwinner of the family, did you receive any help in solving future financial problems?

25. If the patient was a child, was schooling available during rehabilitation?

33. Did you get any help from a social worker or another source in choosing the best rehabilitation facility for the patient?

Most families had to seek information about insurance and legal matters for themselves by calling attorneys or insurance agents. In no instance did a member of the hospital staff, such a social worker, volunteer help with such questions. Even though lawyers and insurance agents recently have been speaking more frequently at support group meetings and seminars concerning head trauma, this participation does not help fill the immediate needs of the stricken family. There is a pressing need for someone on the hospital staff to at least direct families toward the answers they need about these matters in the first days following the patient's admission.

Questions inevitably arise about money to provide the services the patient needs, long range care and rehabilitation, and legal matters. Serious accidents usually involve large settlements, and relatives need to know how to handle such matters, as well as taxes and investments over periods possibly extending over many years. At a time of such great stress it is almost impossible without professional help to anticipate what the situation will be 10 years after the accident.

As with information about legal and insurance matters, families often had to seek outside help to solve financial problems. Wives were left to face financial responsibilities for mortgage payments, food, and clothing with little support. Recently help has been made available through social workers and community agencies, but usually one has to know how to find it without professional assistance.

All too frequently, particularly at a time when it could have been very beneficial, counseling was not available for the patients in the survey. Some received no counseling until the family members intervened, and often that did not happen until rehabilitation had begun. It was common for the patient to feel totally alone and misunderstood; much needless worry and frustration could have been avoided if this aspect of rehabilitation had been dealt with early in the course of events.

Not until recently have support groups begun to form throughout the country to provide counseling for families of victims of head trauma. Relatives often are forced to deal with this traumatic change in their lives by themselves.

In the case of pediatric patients, the question of schooling was not solved, in most cases, until after rehabilitation therapy had begun. Parents usually had to hire a tutor or work with the patient themselves. In recent years, once a child has returned to school, help is made available. However, often in this survey the patient was put into a "special education" class for the retarded. Although modern techniques for teaching the retarded are much more effective than regular classroom instruction, they are not designed to fill the needs of the victim of head trauma. He is singled out as being different, and he feels very much alone. If this teaching could be undertaken by a trained special education teacher who deals solely with head trauma victims, the process of integration into a school society would be greatly simplified. Until recently little has been known about head trauma, and such patients are often thought of as being slow or retarded. It is not recognized that they can think but that their capacity to express themselves is impaired.

Suggestions in regard to choosing the best facility for the patient's rehabilitation were given when family members inquired, but little information was available other than from social workers. Many people had to investigate the facilities available by themselves and make the decision on their own. However, social workers sometimes were very helpful in providing recommendations based on the needs of the patient.

The Patient's Status (Questions 21, 30, 31, 39, 40, 41, 42, 44, and 45)

21. Who was responsible for the greatest progress — the nurses, the therapists, or the family?

30. Who seemed to have the most difficulty in adjusting to the injury — the patient, the parents, children, or siblings?

31. What gave the patient the greatest sense of accomplishment?

39. How did the patient react to physical therapy — positively, negatively, or neutrally?

40. How did the patient react to occupational therapy — positively, negatively, or neutrally?

41. How did the patient react to other types of therapy (e.g., speech, recreational)?

44. Upon discharge from the rehabilitation center, what did the patient do? Returned to work? Returned to school? Had to be retrained for another job? Other?

45. Was there a need for further therapy or counseling after discharge?

To the question "Who was responsible for the greatest progress — the nurses, the therapists, or the family?" the answer was overwhelmingly "the family." Credit was given to both the nursing staff and the therapists, but usually the family's help and support were thought to have been of major importance. Almost all agreed, however, that at least one other person — a nurse, a therapist, a social worker, or a counselor — had also had a significant effect on the patient's progress.

Most commonly the patient was seen as having had the most difficulty in adjusting to the injury. It was apparent that if the patient was able to accept what had happened and adjust to new routines, his parents and siblings had an easier time adjusting.

The survey revealed that the patient's greatest sense of accomplishment was in learning "new" skills. Whether being able to walk again, doing household chores, or simply communicating, each success created a desire to do more. One important source of encouragement was the knowledge that others in the same or worse condition had been able to accomplish the task. Like a child, a patient takes pride in the smallest accomplishment and wants to show off. This trend must be encouraged and used to promote further progress.

For the most part, patients reacted positively to physical therapy mainly because they wanted to get better. Physical limitations made some take a negative attitude because therapy meant pain; others who could not understand what had happened were negative because they were frustrated. Still others, like me, who became children again often slept through therapy or acted disruptively because of frustration, although they might have appeared to others to be angry.

Activities performed in occupational therapy can be fun without being physically taxing. Depending on the therapist, the skills to be mastered can be enjoyable and the sense of accomplishment great.

The reaction to other types of therapy, e.g., speech and recreational therapy, depended on the degree of physical impairment. Frustration was a major factor here too. In many cases speech was noticeably affected, and the impediment distressed the patient and caused him to be ill at ease. Typically, as he improved and gained confidence, therapy sessions became more enjoyable.

When the patient was encouraged by success in one area, he often was able to accomodate to lack of progress in another area. Frustration was the major problem. Like a child, the patient had to be continually encouraged by staff and family to keep trying even when he had temporarily failed.

Following discharge from the rehabilitation unit some returned to work or school and were doing very well at the time of the survey. Many, however, were unable to work because of inability to find a job. Employers need to be educated about the abilities of victims of head trauma. Agencies must be created and training given to help such people re-enter the working world. Although they perhaps will not be able to do the same jobs they did before, they can be retrained successfully for other types of work. I will discuss these matters in more detail in Chapter 11.

Some patients continued to receive therapy as outpatients or in their homes and after discharge frequently needed further therapy or counseling. The necessity for additional counseling or psychiatric care long after discharge from the rehabilitation center is often overlooked during insurance settlements.

Attitudes Toward the Future (Questions 46, 47, 48, and 49)

46. If the head trauma occurred prior to 1984, has the situation changed? If "yes," how?

47. How does the patient feel about his future — positive, negative, or noncommittal?

48. How do you feel about the future — positive, negative, or noncommittal?

49. Would you have benefited from a book about understanding and treating head trauma had it been available when the accident occurred?

Unfortunately there were many negative responses in regard to the future. Even when physical limitations had been overcome, the stigma of brain damage often remained. Fears of being different, being left out, and being alone all tended to make the future look bleak. "Nobody understands what I'm going through" was a frequent complaint. Many were noncommittal because they were afraid to hope, yet did not want to give up hope.

The rapid recent increase in the number of support groups proves that families want to improve future prospects. Families who have joined head trauma support groups have gained a great deal of information about dealing with the effects of head trauma. With this of course comes the realization that much time and energy can be wasted because of misinformation and ignorance. This book is a response to the need revealed by the questionnaire for more information for families of the victims of head trauma.

Improvements and Improvisations (Question 50)

50. Please briefly suggest improvements that should be made or techniques you may have improvised that proved successful and that could help others. If you think of any other questions that would be useful in this survey, please include them here.

The responses from family members to the question concerning improvements and successful improvisations that could help others are invaluable in seeking new ways of treating and understanding head trauma. There was a good deal of similarity among the suggestions offered, further evidence that such patients have much in common.

The need for information was mentioned most often. All the families felt lost and alone, especially in the beginning. They needed answers, but none were available. There were no books or informed personnel to guide them. Whatever is known about head trauma today comes basically from speculation. Professionals admit the lack of knowledge of this nearly unexplored aspect of medical science.

"Sensory stimulation during coma" was another frequent response. This technique seems to be successful in bringing the patient out of coma more quickly. Touching, massaging, range of motion exercises, music, and talking all help in this process.

Counseling is vital for the patient as well as the family. Feelings of guilt, resentment, frustration, anger, and hopelessness can be resolved with proper guidance. This can be accomplished on an individual as well as group basis.

Making the patient feel "normal" is one of the most difficult challenges. Often friends fail to return after a while, and the patient feels an acute loss. There is apt to be little socialization among such patients in the hospital, and they do not realize that many others are similarly afflicted. Not many facilities are devoted exclusively to the care of head trauma patients. Being around geriatric patients and amputees during rehabilitation makes the victim of head trauma feel even more different. Many families responding to the questionnaire suggested using facilities available for the ordinary person, for example, health spas or gymnasiums. This is both socially beneficial and therapeutic.

Response:

In answer to the special needs of the head injury patient, new programs are opening which are devoted solely to the care and rehabilitation of only these patients. Examples of these programs are Meadowbrook Neurologic Care Center and Tangrum Ranch.* Information on these and other head injury programs is available through your local chapter of the National Head Injury Foundation.

—Barbara Zoltan

Trying to "educate the public" seems to be a particularly difficult task. The general public, and particularly employers, should be made aware of the employability of victims of head trauma. Vocational guidance counselors should work as liaisons between patients and employers and accompany prospective employees to interviews. I feel that many victims of head trauma should have the opportunity to teach others similarly afflicted, thereby gaining a sense of accomplishment in addition to the satisfaction of helping others. One important point must be made clear: Victims of head trauma are not retarded. We do have minds, but we need the opportunity to use them.

Another common suggestion evoked by the questionnaire was "Find new ways to help the victim grow." This may be accomplished by starting from the beginning — taking the patient from early childhood and slowly progressing. To cite an analogy, if you are driving along the road and come to a bridge that is washed out, you must either find a path around it or build a new bridge. Similarly, paths in the brain can be rerouted or rebuilt by repetitive training in sensory and cognitive skills.

"Know your rights." When the patient is a child under 21 years of age, the law makes possible many forms of therapy and training. There are also legal avenues that the public does not generally know about that can be used to help families financially and emotionally. The general consensus is that you must fight for these rights even though bureaucratic red tape often gets in the way. One must not be intimidated by either the law or the medical profession.

Another common suggestion was to "think positively." The power of love is an important factor in treatment and recovery, particularly when it comes from the family, but also from the professional staff working with the patient. If the patient is having emotional problems in dealing with his condition, family members may need help to vent their own frustration and to deal with resentment.

---

* Meadowbrook Neurologic Care Center is located at 340 Northlake Drive, San Jose, CA 95117; Tangrum Ranch is located in San Marcus, TX.

Guilt is another major problem. The relative wonders, "Am I doing the right thing? Am I hurting the rest of the family rather than helping the victim?" Often guilt ensues because of an unkind word or thought. One young patient had fought with a brother the day before the accident and the brother had said in anger, "I wish you would die!" When a tragic accident occurs, guilt is inevitable. A woman at the conclusion of an argument angrily ordered her husband to get out of the house. When he ended up drunk and in a nearly fatal collision, she was the one who really suffered. Dealing with such feelings may well require professional help.

All who responded to the survey questionnaire agreed about the importance of home visits. The patient gains a sense of reality, for he has to learn to deal with a nonhospital atmosphere and everyday activities not found in the hospital setting. The family in turn must learn to adjust to the patient's limitations. They have to decide whether they can care adequately for the patient or whether everyone will suffer and thus negate the benefits of his coming home. All too often, when there is severe damage, the patient is not able to function on his own, and one family member takes over, making the patient the center of his attention at the expense of other members of the family. This is another situation in which professional help may be vital.

Here is a common scenario. Ted, 14 years old, has sustained severe physical and mental damage and requires 24 hour care. He has been rehabilitated so that he can walk with leg braces and a walker and can make himself understood to some degree. However, he will always need constant care and will be highly susceptible to infection. His mother has made Ted her sole concern. It was she who had let him ride his bike to school instead of walking the morning he was hit by a car. Her guilt has caused her to be obsessed with his care. Ted has two sisters. Mary, the older, is tired of having to stay home to watch Ted. She has had to turn down dates and her school work is suffering. Kathy, the other sister, is six years old. She complains and is demanding, and her father has become the center of her life. Dad, in the meantime, is spending more time at work and at the local bar because he cannot talk with his wife any more; she is too wrapped up in Ted's needs to consider anyone else's.

In this situation the first question should be, "What is best for Ted?" Full time professional care in a facility designed to meet his needs is one solution, albeit an expensive one. However, a compromise is possible. The mother has to learn to deal with her own guilt and overwhelming sense of responsibility, but she can hire a nurse to allow her time with the rest of the family and to take some of the pressure off her and everyone else.

This example shows some important ways to deal with a difficult situation. The first step is to be realistic. When every effort has been made to accomodate without success, good intentions can be more harmful than helpful. Fortunately this is a "worst possible" scenario. More often there is room for much improvement, and many victims of head trauma go on to live independent productive and fulfilling lives thanks to the love and care of their families. The best results are obtained when all in the family join in the rehabilitation effort and also make time for their own needs.

Money is an important issue. Some families cannot afford such costly care, but social service agencies and other community resources can help. One has to find out what services are available. Even when there is no insurance, federal and local funds can be made available to help cover medical expenses. One should check with the admissions office or a social worker in the hospital. The key is to look for alternatives.

Friends are vital to the patient's recovery. Too often, when there is a personality change in the patient, friends tend to shy away. Families should encourage visits and help friends understand how to accept these changes.

Suggestions for Families

1. Even though the patient is in a coma, talk to him. Play his favorite music. Touch him.

2. Oil and massage his hands, arms, and feet. Use range of motion exercises to keep his joints limber.

3. When the patient has emerged from the coma, play an active role in his therapy.

4. Do not let him see you depressed or disheartened; he needs encouragement and direction. Maintain a positive attitude.

5. Keep a log of visitors and daily events.

6. Encourage friends to visit. Make him feel that he is not different.

7. Encourage him to strive for independence. As with a child, compliment him on his achievements; de-emphasize the negative.

8. Get the patient outside the hospital or rehabilitation unit as often as possible. Just being outside in the fresh air is helpful. Take him home often so that he can feel some sense of security and familiarity.

9. Work with him at his learning development level. If he acts and responds like a child, respond on that level so that he feels comfortable and willing to try.

10. Do not mistakenly regard the patient's behavioral changes as reflecting his attitude toward you. He will probably be angry, depressed, or obnoxious. Remember that his actions are not directed at you personally.

11. Accept help. If a neighbor or friend offers to stay with the patient at home, take advantage of the time to do something for yourself.

12. When the patient returns home on a full time basis, try to carry on as normally as possible. Do not treat him as being different.

13. Let the patient know that you are trying to understand what he is going through.

14. Talk with someone about the patient's problems, preferably a counselor who is familiar with head trauma and its effects.

Conclusion

There are no single answers for every situation. The period of acute care is especially critical because most people do not have the strength and foresight at that time to deal with the unforeseeable future. Legal, financial, and emotional assistance is vital. It is also important to realize that there is no need to feel alone or hopeless.

Families were not the only contributors of suggestions. In the following chapter members of the "silent epidemic" have finally spoken up on their own behalf.

5

The Silent Voice
The Victims' Survey

While working on the previous chapter I was asked by many victims of head trauma to give them a questionnaire also. They were eager to speak out. It seemed that no one else had been interested in hearing their opinions until now. I followed the procedure I used in Chapter 4, going to rehabilitation centers and meetings of head trauma support groups. The questions were designed to be simple in order to get the largest possible number of responses. Some needed help in reading or understanding the questions or in writing answers, but the resulting responses are dramatic.

As in Chapter 4, I will analyze each question and draw conclusions from the information gathered. The sample included approximately 100 victims, some of whom were still in rehabilitation centers. I will also include myself here and relate my own answers to each question. Although the questions were simple, the resulting responses were complex, showing the underlying pain and frustration of this "silent epidemic."

Survey Results

Accident Demographics

1. Was your head injury a result of a motor vehicle accident?

About 90 per cent were. The remainder included such causes as falls from a horse and from a ladder, lack of oxygen during brain surgery, and a war injury.

2. In what year did it happen?

The earliest accident reported was 1944 and the most recent, 1986. The majority occurred within the past six years, mine being one of the older cases.

Victim Profile

3. What is your age now?

The oldest in our sample was in his sixties; the youngest was 13. The typical age, however, was about 22. As expected, most were under 30 years of age.

4. Who was the first person to be notified about the accident?

Usually this was a parent or a spouse. In my case the phone number of a friend was found in my purse. She notified my husband, who immediately came to the hospital.

5. Were you taken to a trauma center?

The majority answered "no" because there was no such thing at the time, or there was not one nearby. Even today in New Jersey, there are only two fully accredited trauma centers: one in Camden and one in Newark. They have to meet a strict set of requirements to be eligible for licensing. I was taken to the closest hospital but had to be transferred immediately because that facility was not equipped with a CAT scanner needed to assess the damage to my brain.

Post-Trauma Recovery

6. Who was the first person you remember seeing?

Usually the answer was a parent or a spouse. Sometimes the only recollection was of "someone in white." For me, there were many strange faces, most often my husband, who continued to come every day whether I wanted him there or not! I did not know him, but after many days his face became familiar.

7. Do you remember anything about the hospital?

Most patients were too disoriented at first to recognize where they were. Since most were in a coma at first, it was a while before they knew what was going on. I do not remember much at all of that time, especially because I had no idea what a hospital was.

8. Did you know why you were in the hospital at first?

As in question 7, most did not know. Because of short term memory loss, many patients had to be told repeatedly where they were.

Residual Effects of Trauma

9. Do you remember events before your head trauma?

The majority remembered prior experiences vividly. My long term memory loss was apparently a rarity. Most patients can remember facts long forgotten by others but cannot remember recent events. Most did not remember the accident itself or the events surrounding it.

10. Do you have trouble with short term memory?

All but a few did or still do. Only a couple of victims were totally unaffected. Even though I have long term memory loss, I do have some trouble with short term memory, and so I compensate by writing "reminders" for myself everywhere. This technique of writing notes or keeping a "memory book" has proved to be helpful in all cases of memory loss. To some it has become a joke. One victim tied a string around her finger; not until she read the note on her refrigerator did she remember what the string was for.

Psychosocial Adjustment

13. What problem was the most difficult for you during rehabilitation?

Answers varied enormously. Many victims found it difficult to accept the fact that things would never be the same. Marriages ended, relationships were strained, and lives were forever disrupted. For those severely injured, walking was the greatest challenge. More often, however, interpersonal relationships suffered the most.

14. Do friends treat you differently now?

For those with severe short term memory loss, the answer "yes." For the most part true friends remained loyal, but the relationship was different. More often pity was the motivation for continuing the friendship. Some family members stayed away from the patient. Acquaintances kept their distance. However, many patients gained new friends through support groups and rehabilitation.

15. Who helped you the most?

The most common answer was "parents." Spouses, counselors, and other family members were also mentioned.

20. Would a book about understanding and treating head trauma be helpful for the families and victims as well as therapists?

Yes, this was a loaded question. As I had hoped, the unanimous response was positive.

Therapy

11. Do you remember physical therapy?

As you may have expected, those who remembered physical therapy were often not happy about it. The memories were painful as was the therapy. Most patients realized that it was a "necessary evil." I was fortunate in that I needed very little physical therapy.

12. Do you remember occupational therapy?

The response here was more positive. For most victims this was remembered and enjoyed. For me occupational therapy varied from fun to frustration. I tried to avoid therapy during the time I did not understand what they wanted from me. When it became a game, I was eager to play.

13. What problem was the most difficult for you during rehabilitation?

The answers to this question dealt with both psychosocial adjustment and therapy.

16. Was there any therapy that was a waste of time?

Those who could remember were mixed in their reactions to this question. Some believed that time was wasted while the therapist tried to evaluate the problems. For example, my occupational therapist wasted much time before she realized that I did not understand her. Some vocational therapy was useless because it was impractical. Many patients could not generalize. A patient might learn to type on a particular brand of typewriter, but could not use the typewriter at his new job. Those with lower cognitive skills could not relate simple tasks to more difficult ones.

17. What therapy did you dislike most?

The answer depended on the patient's physical condition as well as the patient-therapist relationships. The physical therapist got the bulk of the criticism. Today I can see the importance of physical therapy, but during my hospitalization I was not too happy with it.

18. What therapy did you enjoy most?

The occupational therapy and recreational therapy won here, for obvious reasons. The therapists had an easier time with highly motivated patients. When I was enjoying the game, I was highly motivated. I showed off to everyone what I had learned.

19. What therapy was the most useful?

Activities of daily living ranked high as part of occupational therapy. For those who were physically impaired, physical therapy was most useful in making them mobile. Once these problems were overcome, however, working with the brain became the first priority. Powers of cognitive reasoning and interprersonal relationships were also useful areas of treatment. I can see now that all the therapy I received was useful, but it did not go far enough. My brain was untouched by the treatment. What I eventually learned was done on a trial and error basis with the help of my husband, family, and friends without professional guidance.

Comments and Suggestions

21. Please use the remaining space to write any comments or suggestions.

Here I will try to include only suggestions not presented previously. An overwhelming number of patients were plagued by the stigma of being "dumb." I remember always calling myself "dummy." Therefore counselors should deal with this problem of low self-esteem from the beginning. Patients must learn how to deal with ridicule and failure. It is difficult enough under usual circumstances to handle these problems.

The greatest success stories have come from highly motivated victims and families. This motivation must be encouraged. By accentuating the positive gains, the victim feels better about himself and wishes to improve. "Miracle cures" are more than miracles; they are the product of hard work and determination.

Each victim had definite ideas about what should be done in the treatment of head trauma based on their individual experiences. Therefore it is important to have feedback from others so that future problems can be avoided. Newsletters and support groups keep interested persons apprised of current events. These should be encouraged on a national basis.

We often hear rumors of progress in the field of head trauma research in isolated spots across the country, but it does not go much further than that. This information should be made available to the public.

Patient after patient emphasized the desperate need for more facilities, more public inoformation (especially from the business sector), more support groups, and more cooperation from insurance companies, especially when it comes to family counseling. The needs of the head injured are unique though similar to those of the stroke victim. Outdated treatment can no longer be tolerated. Legislation must be enacted to recognize this problem. Public funds must be allocated to research in order to treat this silent epidemic.

6

From All Sides
Family Conflicts

In response to the two questionnaire surveys many family members and victims of head trauma spoke about their problems and how they have tried to deal with them. My husband was eager to speak in behalf of the spouses of victims, and others — including spouses, children, and siblings — were equally eager to be heard. This outcry made me realize that this book would be incomplete without a chapter about family conflicts. Divorce, separation, adultery, family turmoil, and financial disaster are all problems in dealing with head trauma.

My experience with my husband is illustrative. How often I heard, "I know you don't remember, but . . ." How I hated that! Particularly during the first year after the accident, my husband talked a great deal about the past. I did not know that other person I used to be, and I grew weary of hearing about her. It only made me feel more alone. Friends and relatives asked, "Do you remember . . . ?" Maybe they were not pleased with the person I had become. Who was I, anyhow?

Today I can appreciate the turmoil my husband went through. "Why did this happen to me?" must have been his most common thought. He asked himself questions like "What should I do with my life now?" and "How can I resolve these financial problems?" In my "childhood" following the accident my husband became more like a father to me than a spouse. He was my teacher, my protector, my source of security. He put me first in his life, and everything else was of secondary importance. Thus his work suffered, for he took time off to care for me. In the beginning he worried about my being alone, eating properly, dressing properly, and ordinary everyday activities. He would leave work to check up on me, to make sure that I had not gotten into any trouble, which I was likely to do. "I had to take care of my wife," he said — love and obligation intertwined.

My husband, however, found that he was living with a total stranger who did not know him and did not know how to be a wife. He became depressed and despondent. Because of the many emotional and physical burdens, a spouse may lose control of his life. In every case I have seen, counseling is not only advisable, it is necessary; in fact the sponse often needs it more than the patient. I was my husband's first priority; his job was secondary. Frequently employers or customers are sympathetic at first in the face of tragedy, but with time the sympathy wears thin. Businesss is business, and sentimentality does not pay the bills.

The time comes, however, when a spouse must face his responsibilities. When this does not happen, we see instances of divorce or separation. Husbands begin to look elsewhere for comfort and understanding. Even suicide may become an alternative. Marriage and family gradually cease to be important.

Others may wallow in their problems. For the husband who fails in business, the injured wife can become a scapegoat, the "real" reason for failure. "If I hadn't had to take care of you, I could have been a success." Resentment gradually erodes the foundation of the marriage, and counseling becomes the only practical cement that reinforces the structure of the relationship. Once that first year is over, it should be fairly evident how much the patient has improved and what limitations the spouse must learn to accept or reject. If he decides to accept, he must restructure his own life and design a new future for his wife and himself.

There are many financial problems other than the cost of rehabilitation and medical care. Private duty nurses or special equipment may be needed, and legal fees may be a problem. Many families depend on two incomes, and the injury can cause substantial financial loss and put further pressure on the spouse. A husband accustomed to the benefits made possible by his wife's income, for example, may have trouble in making ends meet with only one source of income. This puts a strain not only on the spouse but on the marriage itself.

I had worked throughout my marriage; suddenly that income was gone. My husband, unfortunately, had only two options at the time of my accident — either to take me home or have me "put away" in an institution. There were no rehabilitation centers as we know them today. Everything was done by trial and error. My husband had no support group to call for advice, no one who understood what he was going through. Today he is eager to help anyone who calls because he remembers the loneliness he experienced.

I have benefited greatly from my husband's efforts. However, if asked whether I would have been better off in a rehabilitation center (if it had been available), I now would have to say "yes," basically for my husband's sake. I will never know the answer, but it is interesting to speculate. There is no doubt that support groups and counseling would have made adjusting and accepting easier.

Others have mentioned the same difficulties we faced in our marriage. One husband became overprotective of his wife after her head injury. Although she was slowly improving, short term memory loss made it impossible for her to continue a career as a newspaper columnist. Her husband wrote the column instead, and put her name on the by-line. When she saw the column, she thought that she had written it. His deception left her little room to grow. The fantasy world in which she has been placed has been detrimental to her progress. There are no support groups in that part of the country, and they have not sought counseling. As in my case, everything is being done by trial and error.

Another husband is having difficulty dealing with the personality change in his wife. He has become frustrated and depressed. Having been married for many years, he finds himself now married to a totally different person, one whom he is having difficulty accepting and loving. He desperately needs help and information, but none has been offered, or sought. It is understandable that a person in this situation might seek sexual satisfaction outside the marriage as an escape.

One woman's husband requires 24 hour care. A new wing was added to their house to accomodate his needs, and his wife is often his private duty nurse. Although they go through the motions of a "normal" marriage, going out to movies and dinner, "dancing" in the wheelchair, or socializing, he will never again be a real husband for her. The accident occurred in 1981, and although she still loves her husband, she is greatly saddened by this knowledge. They have learned to cope with the situation, but neither of them accepts it. They feel that they are not the exception but the rule.

Sex is worthy of discussion here because it is such an important part of most marriages. In my case I was a child at first and did not understand the meaning of love and marriage. I would rather have cuddled my teddy bear than spend the night in bed with someone who was a stranger to me. I did grow up, fortunately, and had to learn all over again. Other victims of head trauma are not so fortunate. Some are physically incapable of having sex. For them there are alternatives. There are many techniques for achieving sexual satisfaction regardless of physical limitations. Some, however, may be incapable of understanding what to do. Still others become insatiable, totally preoccupied with sex. Spouses may have to deal with this change, sometimes happily, but more often negatively.

Response:

Adjustment to changes in sexual behavior or roles is as crucial as adjustment in other psychosocial areas. The patient and spouse, boyfriend, or girlfriend should feel comfortable speaking freely about sexual concerns or issues. Although not all professionals will feel comfortable with this, the social worker and psychologist are two team members who have specific training in sexual counseling and are therefore generally good resources. If there is no one available at the facility, the patient or partner should request from the physician the names of community consultants who can provide sexual counseling. Request that the counselor have specific counseling with the head injured population.

—Barbara Zoltan

Drugs may also become a problem. For either spouse, or perhaps both, drugs can provide an escape from reality, a way of coping. There is no one to blame. Likewise alcoholism is prevalent when nothing else seems to help. This possibility alone justifies counseling to find productive alternatives.

So often when there is a drastic personality change, one is faced with the dilemma of learning to love a wholly different person. It is easy to see that this can cause resentment and rejection. The solution is acceptance, but that is easier said than done. That is why head trauma can destroy a marriage and why divorce or separation might become a reasonable solution. If one takes the time to objectively analyze the situation and act intelligently, that might be the best decision, but such a decision should not be made without professional help. Counseling can help put everything into perspective. Compromises and adjustments can be made, but ultimately the solution is what is best for everyone involved. Loveless, bitter marriages are better dissolved than allowed to continue and make life miserable for the entire family.

The family members who most frequently have to deal with head trauma are the parents. The majority of victims are under age 34, and many are teenagers. Not only do parents have to adjust to their child's injury, they also have to deal with the normal changes of adolescence, as well as guilt, overprotectiveness, lack of acceptance, and the resulting marital conflicts and sibling rivalry. As we have seen in several case studies, one parent, usually the mother, does most of the work. Especially when the victim is hospitalizaed, the mother seems to talk over many of the nursing duties.

From the moment of injury, the entire family is thrown into turmoil. Because of the scarcity of information the period of confusion is extended, often for days or weeks, or longer. Lack of sleep, long hours at the hospital, fear, and trying not to fall apart emotionally would drain anyone's energy. Family members can become edgy and emotional so that the smallest matter can cause an argument. Not infrequently injury to a child can result in the breakdown of the relationship, with divorce or separation, alcoholism, and adultery.

If the patient has brothers or sisters, the parents also have to deal with their problems. Later in this chapter I will discuss the particular problems of siblings, but here we see that their problems affect the parents and add strain to their lives. In Chapter 3 we noted that parents had to deal with the guilt and jealousy of their other children. One family insisted that their son quit college to help with his head injured sister, and he virtually gave up his life for her. Not until I told the parents to let him live his own life did they realize what they were doing. Today the brother is back in school and is engaged to be married. Their story has a happy ending because an outsider was there to counsel them. Because they were so involved with their daughter's treatment, they could not objectively see what was happening to their son.

Siblings need reassurance that they have not been forgotten. By following the recommendations at the end of Chapter 4, parents can benefit by taking time out — whether by hiring a nurse or allowing a friend to help — to devote attention to the other members of the family. Parents can help their other children immensely by showing them that they love them just as much and want to devote more time to them. The conflicts of siblings can be reduced greatly with the help of their parents and counseling.

As with the spouses of victims of head trauma, parents face marital problems caused by emotional strain. Often they are too tired for conversation other than about the victim, too tired for sex, or too tired to deal with the other children. The household becomes a battle zone. Family counseling is not a cure-all, but it can be beneficial when all the family members want to work things out.

All these conflicts begin when the victim is first hospitalized, and if not resolved, they can only worsen when the victim returns home. Even if the child is grown, perhaps in college or working and single, the parents may have to bring him back home for rehabilitation. This can create other conflicts. The parents may be accustomed to their privacy, or a sibling may have to give up his room. Thus life styles are disrupted, and new conflicts arise.

Often the problems of siblings are intertwined with those of their parents. Young children, particularly, are not able to understand the seriousness of the situation, the personality changes in the patient, the loss of attention from their parents, and the reactions of their friends. Youngsters easily become jealous of the attention the patient is getting or appalled by the new behavior of a brother or sister.

Typical teenage behavioral changes may be attributed to the head injury. Often parents are too lenient in allowing unacceptable behavior to continue, believing the cause to be the head injury. For example, while I was talking with the mother of a teenage patient, the boy interrupted several times and was not reprimanded. The mother complained that he was very impolite, but she attributed it to personality change caused by the injury. She was surprised when I suggested that perhaps his behavior coincided with his becoming a teenager recently. Teenagers often test their parents in an attempt to grow up and be independent. Once this mother saw that possibility, she no longer allowed her son to interrupt whenever he pleased.

Parents can also help with the friends of the patient. Although they cannot force a former friend to continue visiting, they can explain about the personality changes and the need for understanding. Friends may be driven away if they take the patient's behavior personally. As in one case mentioned in Chapter 3, friends who came to visit a patient spent most of their time playing with his brother. In such a situation the parents may have to step in and speak to both the brother and the friend to let them realize that the patient feels left out.

Those considered least are the children of victims of head trauma. I, for example, have two married children, each of whom reacted differently to my injury. My conversations with the children of patients reveal that reactions run the gamut. Some are very accepting, particularly those who are older and living away from home. My daughter saw me as the same person: I was still her mother and not a stranger occupying her mother's body. She had a family of her own, but she spent many hours with me, and we became friends again. The major changes she saw in me were the childlike behavior and the outspokenness. Other than that, she saw very little difference between the person I was before the accident and the person I am now.

Talking to family members, I am reminded of the story of the five blind men who examine an elephant. When asked to describe the creature before them, each has a different story: It is long and thin; it is long and thick; it is like a tree trunk; it is large and paper-thin; it is smooth and hard. When feeling only one part of the whole, whether it was the tail, the trunk, the foot, the ear, or the tusk, each man got a totally inaccurate picture of the animal. Similarly, several people viewing the same accident will give "eye witness" accounts that make it sound like several different accidents. Likewise, each family member sees the victim from a different viewpoint.

Some children may think that the long term or short term memory loss is an act. If one's previous life was not the happiest, perhaps such a memory loss provides an escape mechanism that the mind creates to protect itself against hurt. Others may take the change in the victim personally. My son quite naturally wanted desperately for me to remember. After all, how could someone forget her own son? Counseling may be the only way to come to terms with these feelings.

As I grow up in this strange, new world, I realize that there are no simple answers. This is not a world of black and white; there are varying shades of gray, which still confuse me. I used to think that I am who I am, and that I must accept that. Yet why do others have trouble doing that? Why do people try to see more than is really there? It would seem natural to want to simplify things, not to make mountains out of molehills.

Research done with the children of victims of head trauma leads me to another important question. Suppose that the victim is living alone and that the child must decide what should be done and where the patient will go. Does that child disrupt his own family by bringing the parent home? It is a hypothetical question that no one I have asked could honestly answer. Here again counseling is necessary to make the best decision for the entire family. The same feelings of responsibility exist for the child of a victim as for the parent. There is no easy answer.

Children living in the same house with their victim parent experience other problems. Some become wild and unmanageable. Some turn to drugs and alcohol. Still others have accepted the responsibility and have become stronger and more self-sufficient. Adversity can bring out the best and the worst in people.

All relatives of victims of head trauma must deal with a totally alien set of experiences that cannot be anticipated. Reactions vary in degree and range according to the individual and the limitations imposed by the injury.

Response:

Family members should be involved in the patient's care early on — not only through observation but in participation. Having the family member learn a task helps the family to understand and accept the patient's deficits and learn how to deal with cognitive, perceptual, and behavioral problems.

Frequently behavioral problems add the most stress to the family. Often patients exhibit aggression and verbal or physical abuse of their loved ones. Behavioral problems are often brought on by the injury. Lack of inhibition from the frontal lobe results in inappropriate behavior, such as lack of social judgment, increased aggressiveness, or exhibition of sexually provocative behavior.

Often behavioral problems are closely linked to cognitive and perceptual problems. A patient forgets what he is doing or what someone has told him. This leads to confusion and confused behavior. If the patient is distractable and has a short attention span he may keep interrupting or changing the topic of conversation. A patient may act out for attention or out of anger and frustration. In many cases it may be helpful to have the patient rest. After head trauma a patient may experience fatigue after concentrating on a task such as dressing or shopping, or when concentrating on a visitor. The patient may need rest or may be physically incapable of any more interaction. As noted by the author, these behaviors may also be normal behaviors relative to the patient's age. Regardless of the cause of inappropriate behaviors, these behaviors must be changed in order for the patient to be accepted into society. When trying to discourage or alter behavior, all people in contact with the patient should provide consistency in responding to such behavior. This gives the patient the consistent message that this behavior is unacceptable.

In response to the physical, cognitive, and behavioral changes in their loved ones, family members may experience emotional feelings such as frustration, guilt, and anger. Often there is conflict with working spouses or parents who need to work and also attend therapies. Perhaps arrangements can be made with the therapists to come in later in the day, in the evening, or on weekends. Problems with distance arise if a better hospital is far from home; does the family send the loved one to the hospital with the better facilities or reputation, or to the one closer to home so that they can visit regularly? Perhaps living arrangements can be made on a short-term basis at the better hospital.

Family members should speak with social workers and psychologists when the patient is in the hospital. Families should also take advantage of the hospital's family education groups or individual counseling. There may also be local support groups available.

Ther are often options for patients in terms of their living situation once they are discharged from the rehabilitation hospital. Private duty nurses, therapists, home health aides, friends, and other family members can come into the home to help alleviate stress and confinement for the family. There are long-term facilities for placement of more disabled patients. Therapy is available at these facilites to further maximize the patient's level of functioning. The patient may be able to return home at a later time. There are also independent living centers in which patients may live by themselves under supervision.

Questions of sexuality and intimacy need to be addressed regardless of the patient's age. These issues are particularly important among sexually active teenagers and young adults. The patient often picks the person he or she is most confortable with — nurse, therapist, social worker, or doctor. Professionals formally trained in sexual counseling and education are often available to interact with the patient and spouse.

—Maria Kendricken

7

Let's Get Physical

The victim of head injury goes through a process of "spontaneous recovery," or natural healing. This takes place during the first six months following the injury and continues for up to two years. During rehabilitation, however, the therapists must enhance and channel this process to help the patient relearn skills or learn ways to compensate for skills that are lost. The emphasis is on correcting the gross incoordination and increasing motor skills for functional mobility. In this chapter I will describe the programs and procedures used in physical therapy (based on information compiled from programs used in the hospitals and rehabilitation centers referred to in the Bibliography).

The progress of therapy depends on the needs of the patient. Therapy must begin immediately, even while the patient is still in a coma. It may be as simple as range of motion exercises and massage combined with speaking to the patient, even though it may seem that he does not respond.

The first step for the physical therapist is to evaluate the patient's physical capacities. Of particular concern are rolling, sitting, standing, position changes, transfers, wheelchair propulsion, joint motion, gross muscle strength, and coordination. Not all these functions can be dealt with in the severely injured or comatose patient. Therefore the therapy given is restricted to what the patient is capable of doing. When the patient is physically able, the therapist is responsible for wheelchair prescriptions and positioning modifications. Wheelchairs are designed for particular needs with the intention of increasing normal muscle tone and decreasing contractures. Correct positioning in the wheelchair will enhance the patient's ability to perceive his external environment with his eyes, use his arms and hands (if possible), and breathe adequately for vocalization.

Another important activity is transfers — moving the patient from the wheelchair to the bed, chair, and toilet. Later the use of a walker, cane, or brace may be necessary to improve balance. The therapist works with the family to show them how to help the patient use this apparatus if necessary.

Depending on the patient's limitations, physical therapy may continue for years after the injury, either on an outpatient basis or in the home. Some patients are fortunate that the need for physical therapy ceases after a brief period, but more often the need continues.

One form of physical therapy originally intended for the treatment of another disease is now being used to treat specific problems common among victims of head trauma. This therapy is called "Neuro-Developmental Treatment" (NDT). Dr. Berta Bobath (a physiotherapist) and her husband (a neurologist) devised this therapy to treat cerebral palsy and other neurological disorders, and this approach is now the basis for the treatment used in many rehabilitation centers. According to Dr. Bobath, cerebral palsy and head injury share two important factors: 1) interference with the normal maturation of the brain, and 2) the presence of abnormal patterns of posture and movement due to release of abnormal postural reflex activity.

When muscles or nerves are totally destroyed there is not much hope. The aim of NDT is to improve postural tone and patterns, but it cannot succeed if structural and irreversible changes in muscles, joints, and soft tissues have already taken place. However, when the problem is abnormal coordination of muscle action (abnormal patterning of muscle function with lack of motor patterns) NDT has proven to be very effective.

The evaluation of the patient's motor deficits is vital to proper treament. Once the problem is diagnosed, treatment can be employed to retrain the disabled muscles. The key is to inhibit the abnormal postural reflex patterns and facilitate normal movement patterns of the head, arms, trunk, legs, and tongue.

First the patient is prepared to move. Next the therapist moves him to develop the normal automatic righting and equilibrium reactions. Next the patient actively moves with the therapist in control. Finally he moves without the therapist's assistance or control.

It is important to keep in mind the holistic concept of the patient — he is a human being with more than just physical problems, so the therapist must deal with more than just correcting a limp or spastic hand. Like other therapies, the physical part of rehabilitation also includes cognitive retraining, counseling, and friendship. A good relationship with the physical therapist can help overcome the frustration, pain, and confusion.

In NDT the therapist treats abnormal postural reflex activity by guiding the victim's responses, as with a young child. By improving postural tone and giving the patient the experience of more normal movements, the therapist tries to enable him to move more normally. The patient is not allowed to perform movements and skills in abnormal ways or with excessive effort. He prepares for functional skills (such as walking, dressing, feeding, writing, and typing) by learning the motor patterns necessary for these activities. For example, the goal is to teach the victim not merely to walk, but to walk smoothly.

The jobs of the occupational therapist and physical therapist overlap in many areas. This is the basic concept of team approach now common throughout the country. This helps avoid confusion and results in the carry-over and reinforcement of skills used in everyday life.

In retrospect, perhaps the preceding information may seem to be obvious, but it is necessary in understanding exactly what is happening. The major problem with families I have contacted is that they do not know what is going on. The changes occurring immediately following trauma are so dramatic and unexpected that family members are constantly, yet needlessly, in a state of confusion. This is a very traumatic time for everyone, and the need for objective, useful, and calming information is great. Often family members see the agitated confused patient and do not understand that his condition may be only temporary. Patience and understanding are the keys to getting through this difficult period.

The physical therapist's ultimate goal is to return the patient to the highest possible level of motor functioning. This level varies, of course, from case to case. For one patient it may involve learning to stand alone. For another it may be learning to sit upright in a wheelchair. And for another it may be learning to play basketball or to bowl. Mastery of higher level skills can be encouraged according to the patient's physical limitations.

The therapist conducts an extensive evaluation of muscle tone, movement, balance, endurance, ability to walk, ability to plan motor movements, strength, and coordination. If the patient needs a wheelchair or leg braces, for example, the therapist can evaluate his needs and work with him accordingly. A program of exercises is developed to improve motor skills. Such training undoubtedly will be tiring and perhaps painful. Physical therapists often are the recipients of verbal abuse and lack of cooperation because the patient is being pushed to the limit of his endurance. He may refuse to cooperate, throw tantrums, or avoid therapy sessions whenever possible.

Because the patient tires easily, the wheelchair is used often, even when he is ambulatory.

Response:
Although a patient may be ambulatory, he may have impaired judgement or be forgetful or confused. He may need to go to another area of the hospital for meals or activities such as whirlpool, pool, or brace clinic. The wheelchair provides a safe, energy-efficient means of transportation.

—Maria Kendricken

The patient needs all the energy he has, and thus he should not stand and walk around throughout therapy. Even though physical therapy deals with the body, the therapist must also be aware of the cognitive aspects of the patient. That is reason enough to use a team approach to treating the head injured victim. The object is to allow the mind to control the body, and that can be done only by dealing with the mind simultaneously.

My Own Experience

I can look back at my "crazy" behavior, the tantrums and the violence, the abusive language and the confusion and understand how I must have affected everyone around me. Because the foregoing information was not known when my accident occurred, my husband and family were in a turmoil over my unexplained behavior. I was fortunate that my injuries were not physical ones, but I needed physical therapy to get my body to cooperate with my mind.

My first experiences with physical therapy were almost comic. I had no idea what the therapist wanted from me, and so I must have appeared stupid or retarded. It was as though yhe therapist was trying to teach a six month old baby to write. She did not realize that I was really a child at that time, and she dealt with me as with an uncooperative adult. Many wasted days passed before she realized that I would repeat only what she did.

If left alone, I would fall asleep. My frustration grew because I could not understand simple instructions. Finally, probably out of desperation, the therapist herself did the task that she wanted me to perform. Once she had done that, I quickly emulated her.

I could not grasp the concept of left and right for many weeks. One day the therapist realized that I was very attached to a teddy bear that was on the left side of the room. As she sat in a chair facing me, she pointed to the bear and said "left." My response was to pick up my chair, turn it so that I was facing in the same direction as the therapist, and point to the bear. Now I understood "left."

Little triumphs like this gave me a great sense of accomplishment and pride. However, there was so much frustration that I tried to avoid physical therapy as much as possible. It was not that my body was not responding to the messages of the brain; my brain did not understand the language, and so there was no response. Although I may have appeared to be angry, I did not know how to express my frustration any other way. I threw tantrums like a child, cursed and fought, hid, or ran away.

Other victims with whom I have spoken also responded negatively. Much of this was because the prospect of physical therapy caused fear because of the pain that is often involved. Particularly when much physical damage has been sustained, the patient equates therapy with pain and discomfort and tries to avoid it. For me, fortunately, there was no pain, just frustration.

The equipment used in physical therapy reminds me of a gymnasium. There are tilt boards, parallel bars, weights, pulleys, and mats. The only evidence of its true purpose in the treatment of physical injuries is the walkers, leg braces, wheelchairs, and canes. The upsetting part for me, even today as I tour rehabilitation centers, is seeing the large number of patients being treated at one time — including amputees and stroke victims. The atmosphere is often too hospital-like. Perhaps it would help to have a spa-like environment. If the therapy had the appearance of fun, patients might not be so loathe to attend therapy sessions.

Evidence of Progress

I am happy to see evidence of much progress in the area of physical therapy. In particular, the team approach has been incorporated in many centers so that all the therapies and the psychology department are working together to help the patient. When all these areas are working as a team, therapy carries over from one discipline to the next and progress is reinforced. For example, an occupational therapist may incorporate techniques used by the physical therapist, and thus the patient learns to generalize. Therapy need not be concerned only with the tasks accomplished in a therapy session; it affects everyday living as well.

Five or six years ago the body was treated quite independently from the mind. Too often the therapy did not seem practical. Over the years rehabilitation specialists have recognized the needs of the victims of head trauma and have adjusted their programs accordingly. More and more hospitals are adding head trauma units, but their progress has been slowed by a lack of communication on a national level. It is my feeling that hospitals and rehabilitation centers should share their findings with other centers so that everyone can benefit.

Many professionals are hesitant to share their discoveries. While I was interviewing several important representatives of various rehabilitation centers, I noted a reluctance in several to share their literature and findings. Not until I began to share some of the insights I had gained in my study did they open up. I was surprised that during one interview the director of a rehabilitation center was not eager to share much inforation about his center's work throughout the first half hour. However, when I began sharing information about the legal complications involved in head trauma as well as innovative techniques being used elsewhere, he suddenly pulled out booklets, handbooks, and other pamphlets explaining his center's program. I assume that the hesitancy was a result of his initial skepticism concerning my motives. Regardless of the reasons, it seems clear to me that communication, understanding, and cooperation could improve the treatment of head injury a great deal.

This chapter is dedicated to those tireless caring physical therapists who go beyond what is required and become friends as well as teachers for their patients. During my interviews with families and victims, certain individuals were singled out as being inspirational in the patient's recovery. For these, physical therapy goes beyond the usual definitions. Fortunate is the patient who comes upon such an individual.

Response:

The physical therapist's first contact with the patient is during the initial evaluation. The evaluation is a comprehensive assessment of specific areas and functions to determine the patient's physical status, identify areas that are normal, and pinpoint deficits that need improvement and will affect overall function.

When the evaluation has been completed a multidisciplinary program is established to meet the needs of the individual patient. Treatment is reinforced from one discipline (team member) to another. The patient is reevaluated on an ongoing basis and the treatment program is adjusted accordingly. The family is part of the team — it's members are instrumental in the implementation of the treatment program. They are able to provide information on interests, lifestyle, activity level, and personality prior to injury, and help to motivate the patient in therapy.

Physical therapy should begin when the patient is in a coma, even when in the Intensive Care Unit. In recent years the importance of beginning therapy as early as possible has become recognized. Therapy can consist of passive moving of joints, sensory stimulation, casting of joints to prevent loss of available range of motion and loss of potential functional use of an extremity, respiratory therapy to maintain clear lungs, and family education and the encouragement of family participation. When appropriate the therapist may get the patient into an upright posture to stimulate awareness and promote physiological benefits such as improved circulation, lung capacity, and weight bearing through joints. In general the therapy is of lesser intensity than that provided in the rehabilitation setting, usually due to medical issues. Once the patient is more medically stable and is moved to a rehabilitation setting, the intensity of therapy is specifically geared to an individual patient's level of functioning (see Chapter 3). The amount of time spent in therapy depends on the patient's medical status, fatigue level, ability to pay attention, and state of agitation. Patient and family goals are incorporated into treatment.

There are a variety of effective techniques used to treat the specific problems that are noted when the patient is evaluated. Some of the areas evaluated by physical therapy, as well as common problems, are discussed below, along with an outline of corresponding techniques currently being used to treat head trauma.

MUSCLE TONE: The therapist evaluates the amount of tension within a muscle in the limbs, neck, and torso. Frequently after a head trauma a patient may have tonal changes which are the direct result of the injury to the brain. The quality and quantity of muscle tone dictates the ease with which a muscle moves.

High tone (spasticity) is an excessive amount of tension that interferes with smooth movement. To the therapist the limb feels resistive and rigid. The patient is unable to control the limb and it may move in a reflex manner such that when a patient yawns or sneezes his arm may move toward his head involuntarily. In addition, the patient's arm or leg may be fixed in a posture, frequently with the elbow bent and hand clenched, or the foot may be turned in and pointing downward. With high tone, inhibitory techniques are used to relax the spastic muscles. Among the variety of techniques used are biofeedback (see epilogue) and maintained heat and ice. For total body relaxation, techniques used include stroking over back muscles, rhythmic rocking, a therapeutic pool, and working in a quiet environment. It has also been found that muscle tone can be directly affected by the position of the limb or torso. The patient is placed in specific positions while in bed or the wheelchair to improve muscle tone. A cast may be fabricated if the tone is too high and the limb will not stay in the relaxing (inhibiting) position. This is a plaster or fiberglass enclosure applied to a joint. The cast may be left on for 3-10 days depending on tha amount of spasticity. Once the cast is removed the amount of relaxation achieved in the limb is assessed. A series of casts may be applied as needed to further relax the limb.

Low tone (flaccidity) is insufficient muscle tension. To the therapist the limb moves too easily and muscles feel floppy. A limb with low tone may feel heavy and be difficult for the patient to move. As a result the patient may need to have his head, body, and limbs supported when upright. Facilitory techniques are used to stimulate a floppy and flaccid muscle to encourage muscles to move. The therapist may quickly stroke over the muscle with ice, a brush, or a vibrator to increase the tone.

NDT directly affects a patient's muscle tone by having the patient bear weight on a limb in a correct posture. This has been found to be effective in normalizing both high and low tone.

MUSCLE STRENGTH IN LIMBS, NECK, AND TORSO: Therapists evaluate muscle strength by giving each muscle a grade according to how much force that muscle can withstand. Because the head trauma patient is often on prolonged bedrest from coma and other medical issues, muscles become weakened and deconditioned from disuse. Muscle bulk may become small (atrophied) as a result of this disuse. Muscle weakness can also be due to damage to a peripheral nerve (a nerve outside of the brain that is in the arm or leg) due to musculoskeletal trauma.

Techniques used to improve muscle strength include the following:

1) The patient may do a series of exercises using weights to strengthen specific muscle groups. Over time the amount weight used and the number of repetitions is increased. Weights are not recommended for patients who have high tone, as often the patient is unable to move correctly and the activity may further increase the abnormal tone.

2) PNF (proprioceptive neuromuscular facilitation) is an exercise technique that incorporates strengthening and facilitation of the limbs. This technique reinforces groups of muscles which normally move together in functional activities. Included in this technique are activities such as rolling, crawling, balancing on hands and knees, kneeling, standing, and walking.

3) Biofeedback may be used to facilitate muscle strength (see epilogue).

4) An isokinetic exerciser may be used to strengthen muscles in the arms or legs. This machine can vary resistance to meet the needs of the patient.

5) When a limb is very weak sling suspension may be used. The limb is held by a suspended sling allowing movement to occur without any friction. The sling fully supports the weight of the limb and allows the limb greatest ease of movement.

RANGE OF MOTION: Each joint in the body has a full available area of movement which is measured in degrees with an instrument called a goniometer. Joints have varying degrees of normal movement (for example, the elbow is totally straight at 0 degrees and totally bent at 150 degrees).

Since many head trauma patients have been in bed for prolonged periods and may have high tone in their muscles, the range of motion of their joints is often limited. It can be improved in a number of ways:

1) Passive range of motion: The therapist moves the limbs through the available range a number of times throughout the day. This is done to prevent shortening of muscles which may lead to a contracture. It can be a means of stretching a muscle once a contracture has developed. Range of motion exercises are essential to patients in coma and patients with excessive high tone or weakness (who are unable to move a body part). The family can be very helpful with ranging the limbs in the evening. Passive range of motion may be painful if a muscle needs to be stretched. The application of heat to allow the muscle to relax prior to ranging may decrease pain.

2) Casting: Once a muscle has shortened and a contracture has developed, more aggressive means of stretching the muscle may be employed. A cast made of plaster or fiberglass can be applied around a limb to maintain the stretched position. Commonly casted joints are the elbow, wrist, knee, and ankle. A series of casts may be needed to achieve optimal range of motion of a joint. The cast is then cut in half, padded, and applied at night to maintain the range at a joint. The family can follow through on nightly application of the cast.

3) Standing Table: This is used to achive stretching of the torso and leg muscles by holding the patient in an erect posture. This allows the patient's body weight to stretch the muscles.

4) Gentle mobilization of the joints to improve a patient's available range of motion may be indicated.

POSTURE: The therapist evaluates if a person can sit or stand with his head, shoulders, and hips in alignment. Weakness, poor balance, abnormal muscle tone, and limited range of motion may still affect posture in the head-injured patient. To improve sitting posture, specific wheelchair positioning is done. This may include using firm inserts for the back and seat, chest straps, lateral supports for the neck and torso, seat belts, wedges to align the legs, and arm boards to support the arms. Many types of wheelchair cushions are available to improve posture while also maintaining skin integrity and ensuring comfort. Specific NDT techniques are used to facilitate alignment of the limbs and torso, thereby achieving more normal posture in sitting and standing.

COORDINATION: The therapist assesses the quality of movements in the body and limbs (i.e., whether movements are shaky, slow, jerky, smooth, rapid, or steady). With an intact nervous system one can perform highly coordinated movements such as tying shoes, clapping, playing sports, and dancing. After head trauma patients often have difficulty planning and performing these activities. Coordination is not necessarily related to muscle strength; patients may have normal strength but have problems with the quality of their movements (such as with ataxia — see glossary). Through detailed evaluation tasks can be broken down into specific steps to determine exactly where the problem lies. Tasks and activities performed to improve coordination begin with simple movements involving one limb and progress to complicated movements involving two limbs (clapping, tapping feet, throwing a ball) or four limbs (dancing, running, performing jumping jacks).

BALANCE: There are two specific balance reactions and movements which a person normally uses to stay upright in sitting and standing positions. The head, limbs, and body react in a specific manner to maintain their upright posture when tilted off balance. The therapist assesses whether these responses are still available to the patient. After neurological trauma, such as head injury, balance is almost always affected. In treatment the therapist works with the patient on maintaining upright posture and will use a series of activities which will help improve balance. Treatment will initially focus on maintaining sitting or standing, first with support and then progressing to balance without support. In standing the patient will progress to activities which require agility, such as skipping, hopping, playing hopscotch, or walking on a modified balance beam that is low to the floor. Equipment such as a large ball or rocking board may be used to facilitate balance and equilibrium reactions. Patients may rely on vision to maintain balance, and it is important to perform some activities with eyes closed.

SENSATION: The therapist evaluates the patient's ability to feel hot versus cold, sharp versus dull, pressure, and touch, as well as their ability to recognize the spatial location of a limb when moved by the therapist, or whether or not the limb is being moved. These tests are performed with eyes closed. If the patient is unable to comprehend or communicate, these areas can still be assessed through clinical observations (i.e., patient does not feel his arm or leg, may get his arm caught in the bedrail, or may not realize his leg has fallen off the legrest). Just as a patient may have absence or dullness of sensation, he may also have hypersensitivity. In treatment the senses are utilized to increase a comatose patient's awareness. This is called sensory stimulation. The therapist may stimulate the senses of smell (by using spices, perfumes, and food), hearing (by talking or playing music), or touch (by rubbing different surfaces over the patient's face or limbs). Gently changing a patient's posture may also provide stimula-

tion. Bearing weight on joints is used to stimulate awareness in patients with sensation problems. Sometimes a mirror is used in treatment as visual compensation for a sensory deficit.

PAIN: In pain is present the therapist evaluates the location, severity, and duration, and how it interferes with function. Discomfort or pain may be associated with a fracture, the stretching of muscles, or severe spasticity. Depression and anxiety can magnify the patient's perception of discomfort. With the help of the physician the therapist determines the cause of the pain and how to best relieve it. Some techniques useful in relieving pain are:

1) Ultrasound: a form of applyinh deep heat to a muscle or joint.

2) Ice pack or ice massage: useful in decreasing the sensation of pain.

3) Transcutaneous Nerve Stimulation (CTNS): mild electrical impulses sent to a body part are thought to block pain impulses from going to the brain.

4) Acupuncture: in conjunction with physical therapy this has been found to be useful in decreasing pain.

ENDURANCE: The therapist evaluates the patient's level of fatigue for an activity. Endurance is almost always affected in some way following head trauma, due to prolonged bedrest, medications, loss of appetite, or injury to the arousal center of the brain (reticular activating system). Therapists gradually increase the patient's endurance by increasing the time spent in therapy, the number of sessions per day, the number of repetitions of an exercise, the length of time a patient sits up or stands up, and the distance walked. The patient may progress to improving aerobic endurance through activities such as jogging, swimming, or using a stationary bike.

ORTHOPEDICS: In conjunction with trauma to the brain, there may also be orthopedic injuries. The therapist stays in close contact with the orthopedic physician regarding precautions and treatment. A fracture, sprain, or strain may present circulatory, swelling, muscle, or joint changes. Swelling may be treated by limb evaluation or application of ice. Mild electrical stimulation to a muscle will assist with pumping fluid out of the swollen extremity. An additional orthopedic problem with the head trauma patient is heterotrophic ossification (increased bone growth in an otherwise non-traumatized joint); this may be suspected in a joint which is swollen and painful and has limited range of motion. It is important that the therapist continues intensive range of motion exercises at the joint to prevent loss of range.

MOBILITY: The therapist evaluates and treats four areas of mobility: Wheelchair mobility, transfers, bed mobility, and ambulation (walking).

1) Wheelchair mobility: The therapist assesses whether the patient can propel and maneuver himself independently throughout his environment on different surfaces. Following specific instructions from the therapist, the patient learns to move in the environment by himself. Many head trauma patients have difficulty propelling a wheelchair secondary to cognitive problems, poor balance, poor coordination of limbs,

weakness, or abnormal muscle tone. If the patient is unable to manually propel himself, a motorized wheelchair may be indicated. A reclining wheelchair is indicated for patients with balance problems, limited range of motion, poor posture, or poor endurance. The therapist assesses the patient's seating needs to enhance wheelchair functioning. Head trauma patints frequently require specific positioning adaptations to the wheelchair for control of the head, torso, or limbs. The therapist is responsible for prescribing a wheelchair that will meet the patient's needs.

2) *Transfers:* The therapist assesses how much assistance is needed for the patient to move safely from one surface to another, and teaches the patient the best way to transfer into and out of bed. If able, the patient is encouraged to do a standing transfer. If the patient is having difficulty, the activity of transferring is broken down into basic steps of coming to the standing position, turning, and sitting slowly from standing. Sometimes a sliding board is needed for patients that are unable to stand due to poor balance, severe weakness, or orthopedic problems. A Hoyer® lift (a hydraulic apparatus which uses a crank-like mechanism to lift and lower) is used with patients who consistently require maximal assistance to transfer. It may be easier for the patient to transfer leading with the sound side if one side is stronger, but it is important for them to learn to transfer to both sides. A patient should be taught to transfer safely to and from the bed, toilet, car, and chair, and be taught the easist method to get up from the floor.

3) *Bed mobility:* The therapist assesses the patient's ability to move in bed. To improve bed mobility the therapist teaches the patient the most efficient and practical methods of lying down, rolling, scooting, and sitting up. If these activities continue to be difficult for the patient by the time of discharge, equipment may be indicated to allow the patient greater independence. A trapeze (a triangle-shaped bar placed above the bed) allows the patient to use his arms to pull up to a sitting position and get his legs off the bed. A hospital bed may be required, allowing the patient to use rails to assist in sitting up or lying down. A hospital bed can also provide assistance to the caretaker in positioning the patient in bed.

AMBULATION: The therapist assesses the patient's ability to walk on different surfaces. For ambulation training the therapist begins with activities preparatory to walking. The therapist breaks down the walking activity into specific steps and analyzes how the patient performs these. The therapist then works on activities to correct the problems noted. These activities are usually done in the parallel bars or in front of a table. The patient and family are often very eager to see the patient walk, but therapists may delay progression to walking while attention is paid to correcting and preventing bad habits. Once a patient is walking, he may need devices such as canes, walkers, or crutches to further help with balance and to conserve energy expenditure. Sometimes a brace is needed to aid weakened muscles in the foot or knee.

It is important to realize that the brace is not necessarily permananent. The therapist should periodically reassess the need for the brace, check the fit, and make sure it is *functioning properly. Walking begins on level surfaces with forward, backward, and sideways progress, and then moves on to turning corners, going around obstacles or crowded spaces, varying the speed of walking, and progressing to ramps, stairs, curbs, and outdoors activities.*

RESPIRATORY STATUS: The therapist evaluates the quality of lung sounds (clear or congested), the expansion of the chest, and the patient's ability to cough and clear the lungs. Respiratory complications may develop as a result of prolonged bedrest or weakened chest muscles (which do not allow the patient to clear the lungs adequately). The physician may order chest therapy following surgery to keep airways and lungs clear or if congestion is noted. Therapy is usually done in bed. In general therapy consists of clapping (percussion) and shaking (vibration) done over the affected areas to loosen congestion. These techniques are followed by deep breathing and coughing exercises. If the patient is unable to cough adequately the therapist may need to use a suction device through the nose, mouth, or tracheotomy site to extract mucous. When exercising it is important that the therapist monitor the patient's breathing. The tendency to hold one's breath when straining or attempting a difficult task is common. To avoid breath holding the therapist will ask the patient to count out loud. With anxious patients using slow, deep breaths aids relaxation of the whole body.

OTHER TECHNIQUES: The physical therapist will note the patient's medical status (pulse, blood pressure, and respiration) and any changes in behavior or physical symptoms (such as increased lethargy, dizziness, headaches, or seizures). Any change is immediately brought to the attention of the physicians and nursing staff. The therapist also reinforces cognitive and perceptual strategies used by other team members.

There are many adjuncts to a physical therapy program. Two which are increasing in popularity are the therapeutic pool and horseback riding. 1) Therapeutic pool: The patient enters a heated pool that is approximately four feet deep using stairs (with assistance if needed) or a hoyer lift. The patient is accompanied in the pool by the therapist. The warmth of the water aids general relaxation of spastic muscles and relieves pain, often allowing improved range of motion of torso or limbs. The water buoyancy can provide assistance in moving weakened muscles or resisistance for strengthening muscles, depending on the patient's position in the water. The pool also helps improve coordination, as movements are smoother in the water. The patient is often able to walk more easily with less balance required due to the buoyancy of the water. Overall endurance is also improved. Equipment such as parallel bars, walkers, platforms, or chairs are available for use in he pool. Patients can be treated individually or in groups.

2) Horseback riding: In this therapy (also known as Hippo therapy) the rhythmical movements of the horse allow for reduction of spasticity. Equilibrium reactions are facilitated and posture, strength, and endurance are enhanced. The patient has the further benefit of being responsible (if able) for the maintenance of the horse (grooming and saddling), enhancing self-esteem and motivation.

TEACHING: Teaching is an integral part of the therapy program, beginning with the evaluation. The physical therapist educates the patient and family regarding head injury and teaches them the safest and easiest methods for achieving maximum functional mobility. These techniques are then reinforced through practice and written instruction. Therapists encourage family attendance and participation in therapy.

(The foregoing section was completed with the aid of Mary Evans, BS, RPT, Specialist in Head Trauma Rehabilitation at New England Rehabilitation Hospital, and Cheryl Kaitz, BS, RPT, Specialist in Head Trauma Rehabilitation at New England Rehabilitation Hospital.)

—Maria Kendricken

8

Get On With Your Life!
Occupational Therapy

To the average person occupational therapy means training a patient to go back to work. In a sense this may be true, but that is like saying that cooking means knowing how to fry an egg; it encompasses only a small area of the total subject. Occupational therapy focuses on increasing the patient's ability to function as independently as possible. The emphasis is on working with or correcting the physical, cognitive, visual, and perceptual disabilities that influence the patient's performance of functional tasks. One of the major goals of the occupational therapist is to help the patient adjust to both symptoms and the general situation in the treatment setting. The patient needs to know why he is in therapy and what is expected.

The goals of rehabilitation for the victim of head trauma generally involve four major areas, although there are others. Most of the data I gathered from hospitals and rehabilitation centers was consistent in stressing the following goals:

1. To achieve integration of cognitive and sensorimotor functions.
2. To be able to respond to an unstructured environment.
3. To be able to participate in productive living.
4. To be reintegrated into society.

Specifically, the occupational therapist tries to facilitate these goals by evaluating the functional assets and deficits with regard to ability to perform self-initiated, purposeful, and productive activity and to assist in developing maximum abilities. Specific objectives are to enable the patient to do the following:

1. Develop perceptual-motor function and sensory integration.
2. Refine sensorimotor systems to provide increased volitional motor control.
3. Increase attention span and activity tolerance.

4. Decrease nonproductive behavior.

5. Develop organization and problem-solving abilities for functional activities.

6. Improve ability areas and learn alternate methods of compensation as necessary and appropriate.

7. Develop independence in self-care, activities of daily living, and homemaking skills.

8. Improve skills for community reentry and educational or vocational placement.

The occupational therapist is invaluable in helping the head injured patient improve. While the occupational therapist does, indeed, treat the patient during coma, once the patient is out of a coma the therapist can judge ability to use fingers and hands (fine motor skills), eye-hand coordination, and "self-care" skills, such as dressing, feeding, grooming, bathing, and personal hygiene. The therapist must evaluate the patient in these areas to establish a total picture of his abilities. By working with the physical therapist (as well as other staff members), the occupational therapist can more adequately assess the patient's needs and design treatment accordingly.

The therapist must repeatedly explain treatment strategies and expectations for emphasis, clarification, and reminder as the patient improves, providing consistency to compensate for changes in moods and abilities. How the information is presented is just as important as the therapy itself.

When the occupational therapist first meets the patient, the groundwork is laid for their relationship. Initially, the patient may experience the following symptoms:

1. Postural dizziness: sensation of dizziness or disorientation caused by change of position or quick movements of the head; dizziness may also result from exertion or fatigue.

2. Headache: intermittent or persistent headache, pain, or feeling of pressure in the head.

3. Fatigue: related to extent and length of time of physical or mental effort during activity.

4. Eye strain: weakness in focus or interpretation due to intensive light, contrasting colors, or movement of visual stimuli.

5. Hypersensitivity to sudden, loud, or multiple noises or movements in the immediate physical area.

The process of evaluation by the occupational therapist involves many areas of concern. The following list is a grouping of specific functional areas which can be used in this assessment. By examining each of these areas, the therapist can structure an effective program to meet the individual needs of the patient.

1. Communication: ability to understand and use speech; ability to communicate needs; speech; writing; gestures; imitation.

2. Behavior: emotional response; self-awareness; appropriateness of behavior; attention; response to testing; type of behavior.

3. Social: awareness of self; awareness of others; appropriateness of behavior; reaction to social stimuli; reaction to family and therapist.

4. Auditory: reception of sound; discrimination; discrepancy of left and right; auditory localization.

5. Visual: acuity; response to visual stimuli; discrimination of size, color, and form; spatial relationships; figure ground; directionality; field neglect; body image and body parts.

6. Sensory: spatial awareness; tactile defensiveness; proprioception; temperature; sharpness and dullness; stereognosis.

7. Physical: passive and active joint range of motion; contractures; deformities; skin integrity; active response; body positioning; abnormal tone (spasticity); strength; hand dominance; developmental level; standing; gait; balance; reflexes.

8. Functional: follow instructions; understand instructions; initiate movement; accomplish task (steps); limitations; deviations; retention; integration; self-care carry-over; presence of deficits in self-care; safety awareness; judgment; level of independence.

9. Educational: premorbid level; ability to learn, retain, and problem-solve; concept and use of concrete and abstract.

10. Vocational: premorbid level and skill areas; expectations; prognosis; adjustments; job situation.

11. Driver Evaluation: visual acuity and perception; auditory and visual perception; reaction time; physical and perceptual physical coordination; range of motion; strength.

Therapy is carried out both in groups and on an individual basis. This may initially involve the use of mats, balls, pegboards, puzzles, and physical movement exercises. Because the patient's performance may be hindered by outside stimuli, the therapist must control bright light, loud or sudden noises, and the distracting sounds of people talking. The patient may have to be isolated completely at first until he can begin to tolerate outside stimuli.

Social awareness, visual tolerance, concentration, and cognitive functioning and adaptation are stimulated by participating in group discussions and activities, listening to the radio, watching TV, playing electronic games, reading books, and reading the newspaper. Learning to adapt to the distractions of unfamiliar environments is important in becoming socially adjusted and independent.

The occupational therapy room reminds one of a kindergarten classroom or an all-purpose room for high school shop courses. Equipment is found throughout the facility. Instructions are given on modified techniques to achieve independence in specific areas. For instance, special equipment like adaptive eating utensils, large print reading material, dressing aids, and adaptive seating devices are employed. With such help patients with various limitations can perform everyday tasks more easily. To illustrate, a woman is able to pull up a zipper with a zipper hook when she would otherwise need assistance; this gives her a sense of accomplishment and independence.

The therapist also can cast the patient's arms or hands to further help him gain coordination and improve motor skills. Assistive devices may also be used to promote independence. Like a child, the patient must first learn gross motor skills before proceeding to more difficult tasks. These early exercises give the patient practice in developing skills. Putting a square peg into a square hole can eventually lead to being able to thread a needle, for example.

When the victim is ready to deal with the realities of his situation, discussions with the therapist may help him to clarify his understanding, make plans, and set goals in adjusting to the changes resulting from the head injury. Working through all the stages of rehabilitation is a physically and mentally tiring process. The therapist can help with patience, understanding, and moral support.

The level of mental tolerance is related to motivation, functional deficits, and the amount of adaptation required to carry out instructions. The victim may display a short attention span, distractibility, or fear of insanity, particularly when blindness, amnesia, or a combination of physical, psychological, and intellectual manifestations are present.

Techniques which increase mental tolerance include relating a task to an interest area (sports, reading, cooking, or puzzles), using repetition in the task to provide practice of specific skills and reinforce methods of performance, and providing feedback. Dealing with these areas in a group setting helps the patient gain a broader focus on social reality, learn coping skills for working with others, and practice assertiveness training for self-confidence.

Following my accident I had no contact with other head injury victims, and therefore felt very much alone. If group therapy had been available at that time, I could have been saved from much anxiety, fear, and confusion. I was unique to everyone around me since there was little public information about head injury.

Functional tasks may then be introduced, including cooking, working with tools, using art materials, swimming, horseback riding, and taking trips into the community (like going to the movies, restaurants, and malls). Often in the occupational therapy room a variety of patients will be working on various tasks to meet their individual needs. The therapist will work with each patient separately while the other patients work on their own tasks. It is obvious that this technique can have some drawbacks. Because of typical staff shortages or overcrowded rehabilitation facilities, patients may not receive all the individual attention they may require. By no means is this the fault of the therapist. Again the reason comes down to dollars and cents.

For some patients occupational therapy seems like a waste of time. To illustrate, Mary (in Chapter 4) had severe short term memory loss as well as visual problems. When she was given instructions by the occupational therapist and then left to perform the tasks, she could not remember what she was supposed to do. She needed continual direction, which could not be provided under the circumstances. It was only with constant repetition and attention that she could complete a given task as simple as reading a sentence.

For many others occupational therapy is the means to relearn or modify skills in order to function more independently. The occupational therapist is involved in the assessment and treatment of a patient's cognitive skills. Although it is sometimes regarded as a separate entity, cognitive retraining often falls in the realm of the occupational therapist. It is a new field of study developed in the last few years, specifically designed to meet the special needs of head injured patients.

To define cognitive retraining, we must first understand the meaning of "cognition." Cognition refers to knowing, awareness, the perception of objects, and the remembering of ideas; it is the learned set of rules by which we think — the rules on which all learning is based. Therefore cognitive retraining is the relearning of methods to compensate for lost skills, based on the abilities and disabilities of the patient. In other words, it is "relearning how to learn."

Each treatment program is unique in regard to the particular patient's limitations. The level of cognition (discussed in Chapter 1) is determined, and a treatment plan is formulated in coordination with other therapies. Continuing evaluation and adjustment are necessary as the patient progresses. In the team approach, now common in most rehabilitation centers, psychiatrists or psychologists and therapists as well as families weekly to discuss the patient's progress.

During these sessions each specialist reports his findings so that each can adjust his therapy to the patient's needs. Family education is important because it is the family that provides support and encouragement for the patient. Initially conferences provide families with information needed in the rehabilitation process. Films may be shown or various problems discussed, at which time family input is beneficial for the staff as well as family members themselves.

Patients are often encouraged to go home on weekends to reinforce therapy and provide a familiar environment with family support. Trips out into the community also help a great deal to familiarize the patient with the outside world. Excursions to shopping malls, sightseeing tours, zoos, or museums help him become integrated back into society.

In the team approach all members of the treatment team are actually involved in the cognitive retraining of the patient. He is prompted by the staff to think, respond, and learn. Among the occupational therapists I interviewed, however, several were the individuals designated to work specifically in this field. The major problems addressed in this area are orientation, memory, concentration, judgment, sequencing, problem solving, and cognitive skills. Computers and video games are often used to help in this retraining at many rehabilitation centers. Some professionals feel that computers and games are impractical in helping the patient to relate to everyday life; others find such devices helpful when their use is directly designed to deal with the specific problems of the head injured. They can be useful in motivating the patient, giving him immediate feedback on his performance. They can be used to focus on specific skills and increased in difficulty as the need arises.

Eventually the patient may need to learn about money management and develop other higher level thinking skills, but at the early stages he can relate more easily to a task that is fun and entertaining as well as educational. I have watched children playing with home computers, and although they may not realize it, they are learning. Memory skills, in particular, are improved with puzzle, maze, and matching games.

Later in therapy prevocational assessment and job simulation are provided in the hope that the patient can return to the work force. Realistic attempts are made to provide a setting for such trainning. Training for a specific job as well as interviewing procedures is given. For example, a potential secretary may work with a typewriter or adding machine, and a carpenter may work with tools designed specifically for his future trade.

Along with this specific training, the head injured person must regain a positive self-image, independence in self-care, physical and mental tolerance, successful social contact and interaction, and acceptable work habits. These are combined with the techniques mentioned previously to help the patient integrate into the working world.

When the cognitive deficits hamper the victim's ability to return to his former job, he may have to learn a new occupation. Aside from specific job training, there are mental adjustments to consider and accept. A former healthy, vigorous athlete may have a difficult time handling a sedentary job, while a former accountant may need help adjusting to becoming a bartender. The healing process is very complex physically, mentally, and emotionally. All aspects of the patient must be considered for the highest degree of rehabilitation.

When the patient is capable, he may be assisted by the occupational therapist as well as a vocational counselor in actually going back to work. This may start out on a part-time basis until the patient is able to work full time. Therefore cooperation is necessary from the business world in providing employment for such patients. The therapist may become a liaison between employers and victims to provide jobs when required.

The vocational counselor often does a lot of the "leg work" for his patients (whether they are in-patients or out-patients). Interviews are arranged, and sometimes the counselor goes along for moral support.

Unfortunately, many victims do not have the benefit of such help. For example, David (mentioned in Chapter 3) must search on his own. There is no person to explain his capabilities or the meaning of his head injury, and therefore he has had to settle for simple temporary jobs like lawn mowing and snow shoveling. David sends out many resumes for prospective jobs, but he naively reports on his head injury; he cannot understand why there are no responses to his applications.

Many hospitals and rehabilitation centers are developing half-way houses to ease the transition from the structured medical setting to private life. Like everything else about head trauama, this is an area that needs further implementation.

The final function of the occupation therapist is to help the patient adapt to environments outside the rehabilitation setting and exercise control over his goals and behavior. It is common for victims of head trauma to maintain the delusion that going home will make everything better. On the other hand, there are those who fear going home because they feel unneeded and unwanted. Here is where the therapist must work with the patient and the family. Discussing problems with the entire family, as well as encouraging group sessions with other families, can make this transition smoother.

Home visits of short duration (one day or weekend) should begin early in treatment. As the family and the victim learn to adjust to the differences between home and the rehabilitation facility, these visits can be extended until the patient can finally return home on a full time basis, continuing to return for outpatient therapy.

Outpatient follow up provides physical and psychological support during this transition period. Through this type of program the patient can gradually learn to adjust to a less structured environment and gain confidence.

During rehabilitation outings into the community can be combined with practice in a controlled setting to teach survival skills. Such skills include crossing streets, using money, finding restrooms, reading menus, ordering food, buying things in a store, paying bills, using a pay phone and telephone book, reading a map, listening to and following directions, organizing appointments, applying for a job, and using a newspaper. All these activities can be practiced during individual and group outings.

To illustrate more concretely what I have said about the therapeutic process, I will describe an actual occurrence that is common when dealing with head trauma.

Fred

Fred was 22 years old. He was severely injured in a car accident. He was treated at a trauma center, arriving in a semicomatose state at about level 3 of cognitive function. Fred was withdrawn and responded only to pain. He tended to turn away from visitors and ignored those who spoke to him. He was able to follow with his eyes some items that passed within his visual field. His responses to verbal commands were inconsistent with what was said. Fred attempted to remove any restraints as well as his feeding tube.

The initial therapy included range of motion exercises and all kinds of sensory stimulation like television, radio, the presentation of odors, visual stimulation, and touch. Fred's overall response to these stimuli was favorable, and he quickly moved into the next level of cognitive functioning, the agitated and confused stage. Here he demonstrated some aggressive and bizarre behavior such as thrashing, attempting to grab visitors and staff, and at times verbally abusing everyone nearby. At times he was able to perform various motor activities on command (like sticking out his tongue or winking), but in general his behavior was nonpurposeful, not at all related to what was going on around him.

Fred had extreme difficulty in relating to his environment and showed increased aggressiveness. He was unable to tolerate a typical therapy program and thus was treated on a one to one basis in an isolated setting. This tended to decrease his general agitation. When the same therapists worked consistently with Fred, his agitation decreased. During this time a behavioral modification program was instituted. This program included positively reinforcing Fred for nonagitated behavior and ignoring his agitated behavior. The resulting behavior was positive. Team meetings allowed staff members to develop a program to keep therapy consistent. This stage, level 4, lasted two or three weeks.

The next stage of cognitive functioning that Fred exhibited was the confused, inappropriate, nonagitated state, level 5. During this period Fred was still somewhat agitated and had to be kept in an isolated environment for therapy sessions. The same clinical staff was used. Because of his lack of attention, it became necessary to present only one stimulus at a time. I have discovered that this can be achieved more easily with the use of headphones to direct the stimulus, which has to be clear and simple in order for the patient to understand.

Information was given to Fred in a logical, step by step manner. The following strategies were also used: giving him messages that were noncomplex and to the point; using gestures to assist him when necessary; communicating with one therapist at a time; and providing sufficient breaks to allow him to process more lengthy commands. Finally direct feedback was given when necessary with regard to his inappropriate responses. It was time for him to understand that aggressive, abusive behavior was not acceptable and was not going to be tolerated.

Because of Fred's mild agitation, confusion, and his wandering from the treatment area, it was necessary to "restrain" him at times. The normal posey or sheet restraint did not work; Fred became more agitated when he was restrained in a traditional manner. Therefore a lap board was used to restrain him as well as serve as a desk. This seemed to calm him down, making him more relaxed and more attentive to therapy.

During this time the staff continually oriented Fred to time and place. A schedule was used to help him identify all daily activities. This was posted on his lap board as well as near his bed, and he was referred to the schedule every morning. Many of his overall responses and verbal abilities were inappropriate, inaccurate, and unintelligible. This stage lasted approximately four weeks.

Fred progressed next to the confused-appropriate stage, level 6, in which he was less agitated and exhibited fewer outbursts. He was still disoriented to time and place but was becoming more aware and even recognized his surroundings. Now Fred was following directions more consistently, and his responses were more appropriate. However, he consistently gave incorrect responses if they required any type of expanded memory skill.

He continued to have trouble in relating new tasks to skills already learned. Use of the daily schedule was quite helpful during this stage, and Fred was more aware of where he was going, what type of therapy was scheduled, and who he was seeing. His therapy was still being given in an isolated room about half the time, but he was gradually exposed to outside stimuli. Initally he did not respond well to this idea of "mainstreaming" but eventually put up with it. His behavioral management program was discontinued because of this improvement.

As he progressed, Fred began questioning about his accident, when he was going home, and what was going on at that time. This development seemed to signal an important breakthrough in his recall and orientation skills. He became able to carry out very easy cognitive, language, and language oriented tasks, as well as other specific tasks, with only minimal assistance. Because his attention span was limited to about five to 10 minutes, it was necessary to continually remind him to keep working on a particular task.

After the second week in this stage, it was decided to send Fred home on a weekend pass. First the family was brought in and counseled regarding the his present state, problems, and progress. Fred went home and returned with family reports of only minimal difficulty. As with every family I interviewed, home visits were positive experiences and the patient was eager to continue therapy with his family.

Fred could tell the difference between his home and the hospital, but he still became mildly confused over specific details. He was able to get through his daily routine in a "robot-like" fashion. Even though a minimal amount of confusion was still present, he no longer needed repetitive commands or the lap board restraint. Fred was able to tolerate therapeutic treatment sessions for up to 20 to 30 minutes. However, it was necessary to change tasks within that short period to avoid lapses in his attention span, boredom, or frustration.

It was also evident that Fred's interest in home was increasing. He now realized that he had had an accident, that he was not "the same as before," and that he was in the hospital and wanted desperately to be home with his family. He consistently repeated questions and statements, seeming to forget that he had said the same thing before. His requests and chatter were seemingly endless.

Fred walked with a jerky and unsteady movement but did not need much help in maintaining his balance or in walking. He continued to have visual field deficits and perceptual deficits, although he was learning to compensate. He required only stand-by assistance for dressing, bathing, and other activities of daily living.

Fred was discharged home after about 13 weeks. He is now receiving outpatient therapy through a home health agency, working with a skilled staff and a psychologist. His family is also attending counseling sessions. Fred was receiving vocational rehabilitation and counseling when he was discharged from the rehabilitation center.

Conclusion

Working with Fred was a challenge and a rewarding experience for all those around him. The occupational therapist, as well as all the others of the team, had her work cut out for her in helping him develop to his full potential. Among the vast number of victims of head trauma, Fred's type of case is often typical, given the proper care. Much of the responsibility of reintroducing him to the "normal" world fell on the occupational therapist's shoulders.

We must not forget the patients who are not success stories. Because of severe damage to the brain, some may never recover their cognitive skills. They may remain forever on level 3 or 4 or anywhere else on the scale. With such patients the therapists face frustration and despair in dealing with the patients and their families every day. However, even slight progress can be very rewarding.

I began to understand how occupational therapists, as well as other professionals dealing with head trauma, find rewards in their work when I spoke with a special education teacher. Most teachers are thrilled when an intelligent student produces a great short story or poem. In the case of brain impaired students, the accomplishments are scaled down to the abilities of the children. Small successes can mean as much as the intelligent student's major accomplishment when seen in perspective. Likewise the small accomplishments of the head injured patient, such as the fixed stare instead of the aimless wandering eyes, or the response of a squeeze to the hand, are truly great accomplishments.

Response:

Although the author has listed several objectives of occupational therapy, I would like to add and expand on the following areas of occupational therapy evaluation and treatment:

1. Functional mobility.

2. Cognitive function.

3. Upper extremity function, isolated control, and coordination.

4. Hand function.

5. Coma intervention, including progressive casting/splinting, wheelchair/bed positioning, oral bulbar (Dysphagia) evaluation and treatment, and controlled sensory stimulation.

6. Community reintegration.

7. Pre-vocational evaluation and treatment.

8. Home visits.

FUNCTIONAL MOBILITY: As mentioned briefly in the physical therapy chapter, one of the goals of treatment is to increase the patient's functional mobility. Depending on the facility, this training may be handled by the occupational therapist, physical therapist, or both. Functional mobility training includes transfer training, bed mobility, and (if appropriate) wheelchair mobility.

Transfer training deals with getting patients in and out of bed, wheelchair, toilet, tub/shower, furniture, and car. The approach that the therapist uses will depend on the patient's status. No matter what the specific technique, the goal is to have the patient become as functional as possible without increasing abnormal tone or reflexes. The family should participate in hands-on transfer training with the therapist so they can feel confident in their transfer abilities before the patient goes on home visits or community outings. If you plan on taking your family member out of the facility and have not been approached by a therapist for training, ask the therapist to work with you in this area.

Bed mobility training includes activities such as rolling, supine/sit and vice versa, and scooting. Again, the techniques used will encourage function without increasing tone. Just as with transfers, it is important for the family to participate in training with the therapist before the patient is discharged.

Wheelchair mobility training begins with propulsion on straight surfaces and progresses to turning, tight spaces, inclines, and ultimately community settings. Training also includes locking and unlocking the wheelchair and removing the legs and armrests. Before the patient is discharged the therapist should also instruct the family in loading the wheelchair into the car.

COGNITIVE FUNCTION: In addition to working on functional organizational and problem solving skills, the occupational therapist will evaluate and treat deficits of attention, memory, initiation, planning, mental flexibility, abstraction, insight, safety awareness, and acalculia. The main difference between the occupational therapist's approach to cognitive deficits and that of other team members is the functional orientation. The occupational therapist, for instance, may work on the patient's deficits related to insight or safety awareness in the kitchen setting. Problem solving and organization skills may be addressed in a community setting (such as the grocery store), while acalculia may be addressed in budgeting or banking activities. Families should talk with the occupational therapist about the treatment approach and how they can reinforce it.

UPPER EXTREMITY FUNCTION: The occupational therapist will work to normalize muscle tone, improve coordination, and facilitate isolated control of the upper extremities. All techniques utilized are geared toward increased functional use. The therapist, for instance, may use positioning and hands-on techniques to encourage development of the hand-to-mouth pattern used to eat. It is important for the family to watch the therapist and get hands-on training when appropriate in order to encourage a consistent approach with the patient. Consistency of approach when working with the head injury patient is crucial.

HAND FUNCTION: As the patient recovers he may begin to show increased hand function. Inevitably there are problems related to weakness, increased tone, and poor isolated control. The occupational therapist will work to decrease these problems and subsequently increase functional grasp and prehension patterns.

The grasp patterns she works to develop include cylindrical grasp (used to pick up items such as a tube of toothpaste) and spherical grasp (used to pick up a ball or other round object). The therapist will work on both grasp and release. Often the patient will be able to grasp objects but have difficulty releasing them. In these cases continued encouragement or practice in grasping objects is NOT beneficial to the patient and in fact may actually hinder progress and ultimately decrease overall function.

In the next stage of hand function treatment the therapist will work to develop and refine prehension patterns. These include lateral pinch (used for turning pages, cards, etc.), three point pinch (used for writing, picking up objects, and the majority of functional tasks), and fingertip prehension or pinch (used for picking up small objects such as straight pins, paperclips, etc.). The final stage of hand function treatment includes actual fine motor manipulation skills and fine finger dexterity.

At all stages of recovery the therapist and family should encourage bilateral tasks. Even the patient with no apparent hand function in one hand should be encouraged to use that hand as a passive functional assist. For example, the affected hand may be placed or positioned to stabilize paper during writing activities.

COMA INTERVENTION: The occupational therapist works with the head injury patient as soon as he is medicallly stable, even if still in coma. The main areas of occupational therapy evaluation and treatment of the comatose or semicomatose patient include progressive casting/splinting, wheelchair and bed positioning, controlled sensory stimulation, and (when appropriate) oral bulbar evaluation and treatment. The occupational therapist may not be the only professional working in these areas of treatment, and in some facilites several of these areas may be handled by the physical therapist or speech pathologist. Who provides the treatment is not crucial. However, it is crucial that the patient receive coma intervention. Unfortunately, there are still many facilities which do not provide this crucial treatment. In these cases it is often the family that must take on the role of therapist, at least in some of these treatment areas.

1) Progressive casting/splinting: Increased muscle tone can become a severe problem, even during coma. Sometimes the patient is not expected to live, and therefore problems such as increased tone are not addressed. As a result, the patient may develop soft tissue contractures and decreased range of motion. Progressive, inhibitive casting is indicated before the contractures worsen. The occupational therapist may cast the elbow with a series of casts which are changed every few days and work to straighten the arm. The physical therapist may cast the knee or foot. In some cases she may cut the cast in half, line and strap it (creating a bi-valved cast), and institute a specific time schedule for wearing of the cast. No matter which method is utilized, the goal is to put the muscles on continuous stretch, thereby causing relaxation and allowing mobility around the joint.

The occupational therapist may also splint the patient's hand, which may tend to flex or close because of the influence of primitive reflexes. The therapist provides a "reflex inhibiting" splint for the hand to counteract this problem. Usually the hand splint will be worn for a few hours (and during the night) and then taken off for one to two hours. It is crucial for the professionals and family to carry through with the recommended splinting schedule. If red marks or irritated areas do not disappear within 10 to 15 minutes, the therapist or nurse must be notified immediately so adjustments to the splint can be made.

2) Wheelchair/bed positioning: Another area of treatment which works to prevent or decrease abnormal tone is bed and wheelchair positioning. Even if the patient is not displaying increased tone, bed positioning should be provided as a preventive measure. Early positioning can prevent or lessen tone problems later in the recovery process. Bed positioning consists of strategically placing a number of pillows around the patient to position him in a reflex inhibiting position. For example, when the patient is in a side lying position a pillow may be placed under the arm and the arm positioned with the shoulder forward and the arm straight. Every patient should receive bed positioning designed to meet his individual needs. The occupational therapist should post bed positioning pictures and instructions for nursing staff and families to follow. The therapist should also train the family in positioning the patient.

Positioning aids for head and postural supports will usually be necessary when the comatose or semi-comatose patient first gets into a wheelchair. Even if the patient is in a semi-comatose state, it is crucial for him to be up in a chair for at least part of the day as tolerated. This will not only prevent the development of lung or respiratory problems, but often will improve the patient's level of awareness. Wheelchair positioning begins at the hips and pelvis. If the patient hyperextends at the hips due to decerebrate posturing or other primitive reflexes, the therapist may provide a "posey lap roll" or padded bar which attaches to the wheelchair and sits across the patient's lap. For some patients an inclined padded seat wedge placed underneath the patient is sufficient for breaking up the extension pattern. Some patients may initially require both. Once the hips and pelvis have been positioned the need for postural or trunk supports is evaluated. Lateral trunk supports or a lap tray may be utilized. The lap tray will also serve as a support for both arms. For lower extremity positioning a foot cast with an inhibitive foot plate or foot wedge may be needed. For upper extremity positioning a lap tray, half-lap tray, or arm trough may be used in conjunction with upper extremity casting or splinting.

Head positioning is the most difficult area of positioning. The head support of a recliner wheelchair may be enough, or at least provide a good base to apply head positioning devices. A bicycle helmet shaped without the outer helmet or a U-shaped device with a strap may be tried by the therapist. Traditional neck collars are not effective and should not be used.

Wheelchair positioning is a dynamic process. The therapist will constantly reevaluate the patient's need for the devices and gradually remove them as the patient progresses. If the patient is not being seen on a daily basis, the family should notify the therapist of any observed change in positioning needs.

3) Oral bulbar function: When appropriate an occupational or physical therapist or a speech pathologist will evaluate the patient's oral bulbar status. The therapist will evaluate oral reflexes, jaw stability, facial sensitivity, and breath support. If necessary she will recommmend a videofluoroscopy (a modified barium swallow) to identify additional problems which cannot be detected from clinical examination.

Having the patient eat orally is often one of the highest priorities for the family. It is often frustrating for families who are unable to see why the patient remains on tube feeding. It is important for families to realize that certain key elements of eating, swallowing, and other areas relating to the patient's oral bulbar status must be functional before it is safe for the patient to eat orally. A patient who is fed too soon is at risk of aspiration. Families should discuss the patient's oral bulbar status with the therapist on an ongoing basis.

4) Sensory stimulation: It is crucial for the low level head injury patient to receive sensory stimulation during the comatose state. Unfortunately, many facilities still are not providing this service; in these cases the family must take on the role of therapist. When providing sensory stimulation, apply the following principles:

A. Apply one stimulus at a time and wait for a response.

B. Use stimulation that means something to the patient (i.e., a favorite record or perfume previously worn).

C. Sensory stimulation should be given for brief sessions with rest periods throughout the day.

D. Use more than one sensory system at a time. For example, talk to the patient while rubbing his arm with a washcloth.

E. Do not provide stimulation of a noxious nature.

F. Do not stimulate with ammonia, menthol, peppermint, or cloves.

Sensory stimulation includes the senses of touch, smell (olfactory), taste (gustatory), hearing (auditory), and seeing (visual).

Touch — Provide tactile stimulation through range of motion, rubbing on cream, and using different textures (i.e., washcloth, leather, velvet, etc.). Provide several repetitions with rest periods in between.

Olfactory — Use perfume, food extracts, spices, etc. for stimulation. Use one scent at a time. Do not mix scents. If possible, use scents that are familiar to the patient.

Gustatory — Due to its close relationship with oral bulbar status, it is not appropriate for families to be involved in gustatory stimulation. Improper technique will cause damage to the patient.

Auditory — Ring a bell, clap hands, shake keys, talk to the patient, etc.

Visual — Use bright and moving objects to try to develop visual attention and visual tracking or scanning.

COMMUNITY REINTEGRATION: As with other areas of Occupational Therapy, community reintegration is based on graded activities. For example, community skills training will actually begin within the facility. It may begin with counting change, making a grocery list, writing checks, or basic budgeting activities. Next the therapist may introduce activities related to the hospital gift shop or cafeteria . When the patient has begun to master these settings the therapist will begin community trips. Once again the progression of settings will be based on the skills required to succeed within each setting. A trip to McDonalds for lunch, for instance, would be less demanding than a trip to the grocery store. The occupational therapist evaluates the influence of physical, visual, perceptual, cognitive, and behavioral deficits on the patient's ability to succeed independently in each setting.

It is often beneficial for the family to accompany the patient and therapist on community outings. The family can then understand what areas to work on and how best to approach the patient after he is discharged. This is also an effective way to begin to deal with social issues, such as having a disabled family member in the community. Often issues such as dependency and role changes will can be dealt with before the patient is discharged.

PRE-VOCATIONAL EVALUATION AND TREATMENT: The occupational therapist provides physical capacity evaluations, standardized job skill evaluations,[1,2] and job evaluation tasks, and also serves as a liaison between the patient and employer, including job site evaluations. The occupational therapist and employer can discuss the patient's deficits and whether they will affect job performance and therefore require adaptation or modification on the employer's part. For example, the occupational therapist can show the employer how to make the patient's work station wheelchair-accessible or less distracting for the patient with cognitive deficits. The occupational therapist can explain that a patient's visual field loss may require placement of materials on a certain area of his desk.

If the patient will not be returning to his previous job, alternative vocational or educational options should be explored. This is when the services of a vocational counselor are required.

HOME VISITS: Home visits by the occupational therapist (or UNA if an occupational therapist's services are unavailable) are crucial to a successful rehabilitation process. During home visits the occupational therapist will identify needs for home modification and ramping. Home modifications may be as simple as lifting a throw rug or lowering a closet rod. Often family members fear that modification needs are extensive, and are pleased when the occupational therapist offers easier, less costly solutions. Family members should not perform any modifications before discussing them with the occupational therapist. This can often save many hours of work and a great deal of money. The final decisions on the type of durable medical equipment (such as tub seats or commodes) should also be made in consultation with the therapist. The therapist will train the family in transfers and mobility within the home setting. Issues such as energy conservation, work simplification, and in-home support services are also discussed at this time.

—Barbara Zoltan

References

1. Tower System: Evaluator's Manual, I.C.D. Rehabilitation and Research Center, New York, 1967.

2. Valpar Component Work Sample Series, Valpar Corporation, Tucson, AZ, 1974-1977.

9

Speech and Recreational Therapy

Although physical and occupational therapy is necessary for the rehabilitation of a head injured patient, the help of other types of therapists is also required in almost all cases. Included in this group are the speech therapist (and speech-language pathologist), the recreational therapist, and the vocational therapist. In most rehabilitation centers these jobs are performed by either the physical or the occupational therapist. These therapies include respiratory therapy, cognitive retraining, educational and vocational rehabilitation, and activity therapy. Using a team approach, these therapies often overlap and are considered parts of other types of therapy.

In Chapters 7 and 8 we saw how physical and occupational therapy helps in rehabilitation. Now we will take a close look first at speech therapy, usually carried out by a speech-language pathology department. We must first understand the distinction between speech and language.

In 1984 the Lake Erie Institute of Rehabilitation printed a booklet which provides the following information concerning speech-language pathology. People often mistakenly believe that speech and language are synonymous. However, there are important differences.

Speech problems are physical problems. Following head injury some patients have difficulty in speaking because of weakness and lack of coordination of the muscles used for the production of speech and voice sounds. Speech may be slurred, imprecise and unintelligible, or absent. The weakness may also be reflected in decreased biting, chewing, swallowing, and eating skills.

Language consists of two aspects: receptive and expressive. Receptive language involves understanding written or spoken information. Expressive language is viewed as the communication of needs, wants, and feelings through writing, verbalizing, and gesturing.

Language disorders occur in many variations. Specific problems include difficulty in understanding spoken and written language, decreased auditory and visual retention span, and reduced word recognition. These are specific receptive language disorders. Expressive language problems can be seen in naming abilities, grammmar, syntax, confused verbalizations, and reduced ability to write or even copy.

The most common problem for a head injured patient is a decrease in cognitive functioning or information processing. In other words the patient has trouble with concentration, judgment, reasoning, and problem solving. Language and speech are tools he must use so that these problems can be dealt with. Communication is a necessary part of life, and it is even more important for the head trauma victim. Feelings of being alone and misunderstood are common and can only be treated when we can communicate with the patient.

Several things must happen in order for communication to occur. These may seem obvious to us, but each must be dealt with to speed recovery:

1. The individual participating in the communication process needs to be alert in order to receive information.

2. He must be able to attend and concentrate.

3. He must be able to remember information in the order presented.

4. He generates, analyzes, and compares thoughts and concepts with previous experiences.

5. Information is then arranged, organized, and related in a meaningful, proper order reflecting the relationship between the individual and his environment.

6. An integration and organizational process follows in which needs, feelings, and wants become words that let others know what the person thinks and feels.

7. After selecting words, a process of programing and translating thoughts into neuromuscular command patterns is sent to the structures that produce speech.

8. Muscle movements are executed that produce speech, and then the communication process occurs.

In cases of head injury one or more of the foregoing steps can be affected. It is the job of the speech therapist to analyze the physical and mental problems and plan a program of treatment. The therapist may recommend other specialists to work with the patient. For instance, when there are hearing deficits, an audiologist may be called in or an ear, nose, and throat specialist may be needed.

Treatment varies with the patient. If the cognitive level is between levels I and III, general sensory stimulation is used. The therapy may consist of the patient's being given simple commands — focusing on objects, turning his head toward noisemakers, touching various objects, or responding to various smells and tastes. As the patient begins to respond, even by a simple nod of the head, the therapist attempts to increase the frequency of responses and establish a simple communication system.

As the patient progresses, skills are increased by presenting structured cognitive tasks in a developmental sequence. Therapy may involve developing the patient's speech, listening, and conversational skills and higher level cognitive skills. It may also include social interaction. In earlier stages, when a weakness in swallowing and eating skills is affecting speech, therapy such as prefeeding, oral stimulation, and feeding programs works to strengthen the oral motor skills necessary for speech.

We assume that swallowing is something one does automatically. However, swallowing disorders (dysphagia) occur frequently in victims of head trauma. It is important, then, for the speech therapist to work with the rehabilitation nursing staff to monitor and assist in feeding the patient. As already noted, everyone must work together and be aware of all the problems faced by the patient. In this way treatment is consistent and is reinforced.

Another area of rehabilitation becomes very necessary when the patient as stabilized. Therapeutic recreation is directed toward developing and rehabilitating the patient to participate in recreation, social, and leisure activities. Previous chapters have demonstrated the substantial problem of social interaction faced by patients. Friends and relatives shy away, and thus new methods of socialization are necessary. There is a great need for more social interaction between head trauma victims who can understand and relate to each other.

Specific skills must be learned at each cognitive level. At lower levels treatment deals with sensory stimulation, activities for increased social responsiveness, basic one-step-structure on-command activities, some reality orientation exercises, and some recall exercises.

At the middle levels the focus is on direct social participation with other victims of head trauma to complete a specific activity. These activities involve physical exercises, emotional and social games, and perceptual skill activities. These activities are all very structured at this level, and once the patient improves, structured activities can be carried out in the community rather than at the rehabilitation center.

At the higher levels the focus is on a return to the home community. Materials such as home phone books, community access guides, local maps, and bus schedules are useful.

Another important service of recreational therapy aids midlevel and higher level patients in participating in leisure activities. For example, game room activities involving ping pong tables, pool tables, VCR's, pinball machines, video games, and stereo equipment can be used. Activities are directed toward those that are commonly found in the outside community.

At this point the recreational therapist's job often may go beyond the bounds of a rehabilitation facility. She may assume the role of "public relations person" by introducing the patient to the outside world, a job also done by occupational therapists. The therapist may also be a "social director," organizing dances and other social events for the patients.

There is one other form of therapy that many facilities now have as a separate entity, although the job is still often done by occupational therapy departments. The vocational therapist works with patients at higher cognitive levels who are ready to work in the outside community. This therapy involves more than just training for a particular job. It includes improving the patient's social skills as well as working with the business sector to promote understanding and willingness to hire a head injured patient. The therapist often becomes a friend, a link between the rehabilitation atmosphere and the real world. Vocational therapy, then, is another "public relations" job, requiring ingenuity and determination as well as skill.

It is obvious that treating head trauma is not a simple matter. Many types of therapy are involved. However, as we shall see next, there is a "mixed bag" of professionals who work with the patients at all or at various stages of recovery. I have devoted an entire chapter to this catch-all category because these are usually the "behind the scenes" people, the "unsung heroes" who examine, organize, and implement the programs necessary for treatment.

10

Unsung Heroes
Other Therapies

The complexities of treatment in head trauma require the services of a wide spectrum of professionals that the average person rarely imagines exists. Among them are neuropsychologists, psychiatrists, cognitive retrainers, facilitators, and rehabilitation nurses, as well as representatives of numerous other related occupations. In the course of my extensive interviewing of professionals in each of these fields, I learned a great deal that I would like to share with the reader. Even though I was a victim of head trauma, I was relatively ignorant of what was going on around me at the time of my hospitalization. My study has opened my eyes to the progress made over the past several years as well as the deficiencies of our present systems.

In my research I came across much useful information in books on subjects other than head trauma (including a text on "Abnormal Psychology" quoted below). In one book, for example, I learned that stroke victims are being treated with techniques very similar if not identical to those used in treating head injuries. I also found data in conference pamphlets, hospital leaflets, and journal artciles. One of the contributors to this book, Barbara Zoltan, MA, OTR, has written a book with Ellen Siev and Brenda Freishtat entitled *Perceptual and Cognitive Dysfunction in the Adult Stroke Patient* (Slack, Inc., 1986). I have paraphrased some information from that book here (particularly in chapters 8 and 10) to inform the reader about what is being done in the field of cognitive dysfunction as it relates to head injury.

One of my purposes in writing this book was to gather useful information for the reader into a handy reference; this will save valuable time otherwise spent searching through a lot of redundant or perhaps inaccurate data. The tests described later in this chapter are mostly standardized. The evaluations and treatments described have been either paraphrased for simplicity or directly quoted.

A Look At The Past

I decided to find out what was known about head injury 20 to 30 years ago and was fascinated to compare what was known then with what we know today. It was as though I had traveled in a time machine. I would like to present my findings, analyze our progress, and then submit my prognosis of where we will be 20 years from now. My source of information is a college textbook used in the mid 1960s for abnormal psychology classes. It was first printed in 1948, with the last known reprint in 1964. *The Abnormal Personality* was written by a Harvard clinical psychologist, Dr. Robert W. White.

Head Trauma

In a chapter entitled "Effects of Injuries and Abnormal Conditions of the Brain," under the heading of "Varieties of Pathological Process," are revealing paragraphs about what was then known about head trauma. In the following discussion each relevant paragraph from that book is followed by my interpretation based on today's knowledge:

"Next on the list of cerebral mishaps is trauma, some direct physical injury to brain tissue. The head and the underlying cerebral tissue may be traumatized at the time of birth if the labor is extremely prolonged and difficult, so that the head is exposed to severe pressure. Any severe blow on the head may produce swelling and injury of brain tissue. Most children, of course, fall on their heads from time to time without damage, but occasionally some of these accidents produce temporary and even permanent brain injury. If the skull is fractured, and especially if brain tissue is penetrated as is the case in bullet or shrapnel wounds, a marked change in mental performance may result. Even when the wounds heal there may be atrophy and scar formation in the brain which impair its normal functioning. Another form of direct injury is caused by cerebral tumors. As a tumor grows, it crowds and distorts the surrounding brain tissue. Up to a certain point, especially if the growth is slow, the brain tissue can adapt itself to the change without functional impairment, but eventually the crowding prevents normal metabolism in the nerve cells."

I find a serious omission from this paragraph, i.e., the injury that occurs to the brain when there is no fracture or head wound (a "closed" head injury). There is no mention of the damage from vibration of the brain within the skull due to a blow to the head.

Although the information presented here is mostly true today, it falls short of the whole truth.

Some of the patients responding to my questionnaire had sustained gunshot and shrapnel wounds, and their behavior was indicative of head trauma. However, this form of injury now constitutes only a small proportion of the total number of head injuries. Furthermore, today patients with brain tumors are dealt with separately, and surgery may be effective in their treatment.

"In war and in civilian accidents the brain is sometimes the site of direct physical injury. This injury is chiefly to the cerebral cortex, which lies directly beneath the skull, although it may reach the thalamus and lower brain centers as well. Occasionally the cortex is the site of disease such as brain tumor or a degenerative process, so that parts of the tissue have to be surgically removed. These accidents and interventions are the source of such information as we have about the functions of the human brain. From the point of view of scientific research, the situation is far from ideal. The scientist can seize such opportunities as are offered him by the heartless course of events, but he cannot create the experimental conditions that might help himn to answer crucial questions. Our knowledge of the brain, in spite of a large amount of research, is still very limited; and the interpretation of what goes on remains quite speculative."

This paragraph sends chills down my spine! Obviously the only way we found out anything in those days was through autopsy. Nothing was known about the treatment of head injured patients and what could be learned from working with them. And to think that the only apparent solution was to operate! This sounds more like medieval medicine than "modern" science.

Another thought comes to mind. If professionals at that time were willing to admit that many of their ideas were speculative, why do they appear to have been so rigid in their diagnosis of brain related problems? I got the impression that their treatments were at that time the only way of handling the situation.

Localization of Cortical Function

"One possible idea about the cerebral cortex would be that each bit of it governed some particular process or activity. We know that in the spinal cord there is clear localization of this kind, and that in lower brain structures such as the medulla, cerebellum, and thalamus it has been possible to find centers for fairly specific functions. In 1861 the French surgeon Broca made a discovery that suggested precise localization in the cortex itself. He had the opportunity to examine carefully and later to do an autopsy on a patient who for many years had been unable to speak. There were no defects in the muscles involved in speech, and the patient could communicate by signs in a way that indicated unimpaired intelligence. The autopsy showed a small circumscribed lesion, apparently of long standing, in the left cerebral hemisphere. This led Broca to conclude that he had located the center for speech. His discovery inspired subsequent investigators to try to map the functions of the rest of the cortex. Most of the research was done with animals, but there were occasional opportunities to make parallel observations with human subjects. On the whole the results have not been what Broca would have expected. Some areas, to be sure, have a certain specificity. It can be predicted, for instance, that injury to the occipital poles, at the very back of the head, will cause an interference with visual functions but not affect auditory or motor processes. Similarly, injury to the temporal lobes, in the temples, is likely to affect auditory function but leave vision undisturbed. The largest part of the cortex, however, seems to have very little specificity of function, and its injury has often produced fewer identifiable consequences than might have been expected."

Today the ways in which the brain works, although still somewhat of a mystery, are better understood. For instance we know now that the cortex is divided into four "lobes," each having specialized functions and skills:

1. Frontal lobe: emotional control, motivation, social functioning, expressive language, inhibition of impulses, motor integration, and voluntary movement.

2. Temporal lobe: memory, receptive language, sequencing, and musical awareness.

3. Parietal lobe: sensation, academic skills such as reading, and awareness of spatial relationships.

4. Occipital lobe: visual perception.

We also know that the cortex is divided into two hemispheres. The dominant hemisphere (usually the left) controls verbal functions (speaking, writing, reading, calculating), whereas the right hemisphere generally controls functions that are more visual-spatial in nature (visual memory, copying, drawing, rhythm).

Although the areas of the brain were known in the 1960s, their exact functions were speculative. Through sophisticated techniques today, using electrodes and modern equipment, we can more accurately identify what part of the brain controls what function. Twenty to 25 years ago autopsy was the only means of study.

A common problem in head injury — damage to the brain stem — was virtually unheard of in the 1960s. Brain stem damage was apparently treated like other kinds of brain damage. Retraining was given on a trial and error basis, and it appeared to be sheer luck that some patients responded positively.

"Findings of this kind have led some workers to believe that the functions of the cerebral cortex are of a highly general nature. In the most radical form of this theory, it is claimed that the various parts are largely equipotential: defects will be in proportion to the amount of tissue that is damaged, more or less regardless of its location. In effect this assigns to the cortex a generalized organizing power, leaving to lower centers the specifics of what is to be organized. Comparing the two views, the student will recognize one of those situations where the truth is more likely to lie somewhere in the middle than at either extreme. There is certainly some localization in the cortex, but it is equally certain that we would miss important information if we were not alert to the general consequences of abnormal conditions in the brain."

I reread this paragraph many times only to realize that it was a mass of conjecture with no substantiating fact. I wonder how psychologists at that time would have explained how some head injured patients could be retaught certain skills even though the center for those skills was destroyed. You will read later about a man who relearned how to read using other parts of his brain, but no explanation is given. The huge gaps in understanding were evident everywhere. Fortunately those gaps are closing and leave me with a very optimistic feeling about the future of psychology.

The two views just presented are poorly differentiated. According to one viewpoint very specific functions were assigned to various parts of the brain; damage to one area was irreparable. In the other view, functions were very generalized, and damage depended on the amount of brain tissue destroyed. In other words, damage to the brain by injury seemed to be more easily corrected because other areas of the brain could compensate for the damage. Both viewpoints are indeed extreme, and we now realize that a compromise is indeed the case. All this, however, was purely supposition 20 or 30 years ago.

"We shall consider first the effects that seem to be closely connected with location. The cortex has been mapped by Brodman into 46 areas distinguished by the architecture of the cell layers. Part of this scheme is represented by the numbers on the accompanying figure which shows the left cerebral hemisphere as it would be seen from the left side. These structurally different areas, however, correspond in only a few cases to areas having known specific functions. The diversity of architecture is not matched by diversity of functions.

"The main sensory receiving stations in the cortex occupy a relatively small space. Area 17 is the center for vision, area 41 for hearing, areas 1, 2, 3, and 5 for touch and pressure from skin and deep end organs. The areas immediately surrounding these centers probably have a somewhat restricted function; area 18, for instance, is believed to be limited to the perceptual elaboration of visual impressions. Area 4 is the motor area which when stimulated gives rise to specific muscular movements, and area 6 seems closely related to the motor sphere. This is about as far as one can go with specific localizations. Of the remainig parts of the cortex, two large zones are of particular interest. One of these is the frontal area, represented by the numbers 9, 10, 11, and possibly 45. It is the elaborate development of the frontal cortex that gives man his high forehead and intelligent appearance in comparison with chimpanzees and monkeys, so that in popular thought the frontal areas are associated with the distinctively human attainments. The other area, the parietotemporal, represented on the diagram by the numbers 39, 40, 42, 43, and 44, turns out in fact to bear a special relation to the distinctively human attainments of language and the meaning of symbols. Curiously enough, this complex array of skills is dependent only on the leading or dominant hemisphere, the left in right-handed and the right in left-handed people. Injury to the parietotemporal area in the dominant hemisphere is a disaster. Injury to the corresponding area in the other hemisphere has somewhat less serious consequences, having no effect, for instance, on language. To this extent there is localization of function between the two hemispheres. Research on penetrating head wounds indicates that the areas in the left hemisphere governing the right hand do not exactly correspond to the areas in the right hemisphere contolling the left hand, which suggests that the whole organization of the two sides of the brain may be different."

This information shows us that the psychologists of the 1960s were heading in the right direction although their knowledge was sketchy. Today we know that damage to one side of the brain, particularly in a younger person, can be compensated for by relearning using the opposite hemisphere. We know that a large percentage of the brain is unused; therefore the potential for learning or relearning is vast. This is one area where I can see great advances, even though research and experimentation tell us that there is much left to learn.

I found a close relationship between what was known in the 1860s and what was known 100 years later. Until the time of Broca almost nothing was known about the functions of the brain. The only treatment was placement in a mental institution. I had the opportunity to discuss this problem with someone who visited a mental institution in 1964 as part of a college psychology class. Her observations were startling and depressing. The treatment in this "modern" facility was no different from what it had been 100 years before. Although clinical psychologists were desperately trying to understand their patients, they were lost. Brain injured patients were mixed into a population of manic-depressives, schizophrenics, and other truly "insane" patients. Little wonder that head injury was a "silent epidemic." It could not be heard over the screams of insanity.

Aphasia

"Injury to the parietotemporal area in the dominant hemisphere produces an effect chiefly on language. This area lies between the centers for vision, the centers for hearing, and the motor centers. The use of language involves vision (apprehending the written word), hearing (apprehending the spoken word), and the motor acts of speaking and writing. It is not surprising, therefore, that injury of the parietotemporal cortex disturbs the language function in one way or another. The resulting conditions are known by the general name of aphasia."

Insight into the causes and treatment of aphasia was fairly advanced. The groundwork was laid for present-day treatment that has proved to be very effective. The following two paragraphs further expand on this knowledge:

"The results of injury are extremely complex. At first sight the disorders seem highly selective and highly restricted. Thus one patient may display only an inability to read, his understanding of spoken language and his speech and writing being uninjured. Another may have a specific inability to find words, especially nouns, to express the thoughts he has in mind. Such a patient may show by gestures and fragments of speech that he remembers perfectly the details of a walk he has just taken, but he is unable to bring out the proper words to describe the objects he has seen along the way.

"These reflections make it possible to grasp more clearly the process of recovery from aphasia. Good results are often obtained by the process of retraining. Sometimes a portion of language behavior is gone beyond repair, so that it is necessary to teach the patient some roundabout method of overcoming the defect. This is illustrated in a case reported by Gelb and Goldstein, in which the patient had become unable to recognize any objects through visual experience. It was impossible to retrain his visual recognition, but he learned to read again by a combination of eye movements and finger movements. He traced the letters with his fingers and followed them with his eyes, providing himself in this way with the cues necessary for recognition. More typically, however, retraining does not involve new learning; it involves the reappearance of old learning which had been suppressed by the injury. It may take a long time to bring about some use of the suppressed function, but once it has begun to operate again it may soon be restored as a whole."

Here would be the perfect place to insert information about long term and short term memory loss, but significantly it is missing. I did not even find the terminology mentioned or any symptoms discussed that would relate to this problem. Although the information given hints at some memory disorders, it is lacking in scope. Nonetheless the techniques then used for relearning — the cuing and the repetition — are still used effectively today in dealing with aphasia.

Cognitive Functioning

"Although the brain-injured patient is inclined to be apathetic rather than excited, it is possible to detect certain similarities between his general impairments and those seen in delirious patients. Overinclusion, for instance, is highly characteristic of the brain-injured, who are readily distracted by external impressions, and a fragmentation of behavior is often the consequence. Probably we can assume that there is a similar difficulty in maintaining directive attitudes, but the wild disorder of delirious behavior is counterbalanced in the brain-injured by a tendency toward rigid perseveration. Attention sometimes becomes riveted on some object of interest, and if the patient manages to solve some difficult problem he keeps trying to repeat this solution on new tasks."

At the time this text was written nothing was known about levels of cognitive functioning. We know now that the excited, confused stage is often temporary, and its treatment is related to the cognitive level. One cannot hope to treat a patient at level III, for example, as one would a delirious patient; the therapy would be totally ineffective. Similarities were also drawn between head injury and other disorders. However, there apparently was no understanding that the behavior of head injured patients differs significantly at various levels of cognitive functioning and that the treatment cannot be the same in all cases. Today we have a similar problem with head injured patients and stroke victims; although the characteristics of both are often parallel, there are differences that require individualization of treatment.

Figure-Ground Disorders

"Many workers attach considerable importance to another consequence of cerebral injury. This is described as a blurring of the boundaries between figure and ground. It is very obvious in normal perception, especially visual perception, that a certain portion of what is perceived constitutes a clearly defined figure, the remainder being a less clearly defined ground. In certain ambiguously drawn pictures it is possible to make figure and ground reverse themselves in rapid succession, but ordinarily the two can be clearly discriminated. This characteristic of perception applies also to any complex process in the nervous system. An action such as raising the arm constitutes figure, but is accompanied by a ground of readjustments in other muscles which keep the body in equilibrium. In brain injury, then, especially in injury to the cortex, the relation of figure and ground is disturbed and leveled."

This figure-ground disorder is treated at present by such techniques as sensory integration, described in the Epilogue. The occupational therapist is trained to deal with these specific problems. The patient's concept of his physical self in relationship to his environment can be improved through techniques designed to overcome these figure-ground deficiencies. The prospects for future treatment in these disorders are very positive as the work of these therapists with their head injured patients continues. Patterns of response can be predicted and adjusted through effective therapy.

Cognitive retraining is also effective in dealing with this problem. Through one's mental processes, physical relationships can be analyzed and understood. Thus, a combination of techniques would seem to be the ultimate successful treatment. That, alone, is evidence of the effectiveness of a team approach to the treatment of head injuries.

The Ability to Abstract

"Goldstein has attempted to conceptualize the most important general consequence of brain injury as a loss of the abstract attitude. . . .It is not an acquired mental set or even a specific aptitude. It is rather 'a capacity level of the total personality.' In contrast to the concrete attitude, which is realistic, immediate, and unreflective, the abstract attitude includes in its scope more than the immediately given situation. The real stimulus is transcended and dealt with in a conceptual fashion. Objects before us are seen as members of a class or category, or they are apprehended in a framework of wider implications. To take a very simple example: a patient shows great skill in throwing balls into boxes that are located at different distances from him, but he is unable to say which box is farthest away or how he manages to aim differently. He is able to function concretely but not to manage the abstract idea of distance, and he can give no account of throwing harder or less hard. Another patient can count numbers on his fingers and in other roundabout ways, coming out with results that look like good arithmetic, but he cannot state where 7 is more or less than 4. The importance of loss of the abstract attitude becomes even clearer when we consider the following limitations: the patient cannot keep in mind several aspects of a situation at one time, cannot readily grasp the essentials of a given whole, cannot plan his actions ahead in ideational fashion."

This paragraph is really the inspiration for the advances in cognitive retraining. Although at first it may appear to be a mass of technical double-talk, the main idea is quite clear: reasoning and understanding are primary considerations in treating the patient. If he cannot think abstractly, he will have difficulty in resuming a "normal" life. We know that other areas of the brain can take over the functions of damaged areas to a degree, and through retraining and education we are learning to deal with the aforementioned problems. There are now specific tasks and skills that help develop the patient's ability to think and reason. These techniques have the potential, over the next one or two decades, of working wonders in this area. The results to date have been very encouraging, and the more experience that is gained, the more likely it is that techniques will be further refined and simplified to produce even more spectacular results.

Agitation

"Brain injury makes it difficult to deal with anything that is unexpected. It is frequently observed that the patients start violently when they are addressed. One means of protection against sudden irritations of this kind is to be constantly busy."

Today we have other methods of dealing with this problem. It is important to realize that this agitated state is often just a level of cognitive functioning that will be outgrown as the patient improves. It would seem that creating a peaceful atmosphere would be more effective in dealing with the patient's fears. It is difficult to remain busy when there is a serious problem with short term memory loss or limited attention span.

"Children with a history of head trauma or encephalitis often showed, along with an abnormal EEG, marked restlessness, emotional instability, and difficulty in accepting the restraints of socialized living. From studies we have just learned that brain-injured children display several distinct peculiarities, notably a ready distractibility, a blurring of figure-ground organization, and an incapacity for the abstract attitude. The behavioral peculiarites of these children are closely related to their mental peculiarities. It has often been noted, for example, that they tend to be inconsiderate of the rights and feeling of others. If brain injury renders a child incapable of taking the abstract attitude, it also makes him virtually incapable of being considerate of others. His failure to become a socialized member of groups comes partly from an intellectual inability to grasp what it means to be a considerate group member."

Here there is some understanding, but again the discussion does not go far enough. I cannot help but relate this to several of my case studies of teenagers who became inconsiderate after their accidents. Perhaps typical teenage behavior is appearing in these cases as well as the unknown effect of peer pressure. If a child is teased and humiliated because of the obvious symptoms of injury, his behavior may change accordingly. The foregoing paragraph may be correct to a point, but it omits other important possibilities.

Attitudes Toward Family and Friends

The preceding quotation also points out a serious omission that is of utmost importance today — the effect of brain injury on family and friends. In none of my research into the treatment of the head injured in the 1960s did I come across any mention of how anyone other than the victim reacted. Present-day recognition of head injury as a unique entity has enhanced concern for those who love the patient. Since most patients in earlier decades were institutionalized or hidden away, the family response was like that of those dealing with an insane family member. Although it was painful to admit, the "sick" relative was put away and almost forgotten.

Amnesia

Another important consideration in relation to head injury is especially familiar to me. It is difficult now to appreciate how little was known in 1964 about amnesia. I suppose that 20 years from now investigators will look back at the 1980s and note how archaic our thinking was, just as we look back at our recent past.

In those days the association of amnesia with head injury was not even mentioned. It was studied in relation to alcoholism, epilepsy, and general paralysis. There was no hint of a relationship between head injury and the loss of memory or a distinction between long term and short term memory loss.

"We turn now to a group of disorders generally classed with hysteria, but characterized by peculiarities especially in the realm of memory. Whether we are dealing with a brief amnesia, a more extended fugue, or a fully developed double or multiple personality, the central feature of the disorder is a loss of personal identity. The patient forgets who he is and where he lives. He loses the symbols of his identity and also the memories of his previous life that support a continuing sense of selfhood. The phenomenon is familiar through newspaper reports of cases of amnesia. Perhaps the patient is so confused by the loss of memory that he approaches a police officer to ask for help. In other cases — these are the ones technically called fugues — he may go on for quite a while functioning as an adequate new person, perhaps with a new name. There are reports of cases in which a patient has remained in a fugue state for months and even years. Conceivably, such a change might be permanent, but we would have no access to such cases.

"It is a little unfortunate that the term amnesia has been captured by the press for just this particular type of memory disorder. Literally, amnesia means any kind of pathological forgetting, whether caused by drugs, brain injuries, old age, or psychogenic factors. The cases we are considering here represent a particular type of amnesia, the forgetting of personal identity. This particular pattern seems to be wholly psychological in character. The forgetting is somehow connected with neurotic conflict and represents an attempt to do something about that conflict."

Strange, is it not, that although the definition herein mentions brain injury, amnesia was considered to be a purely psychological disorder. There is no mention of the possible anatomical damage and physiological changes that may have caused the amnesia. I shudder when I think what might have happened to me had my accident occurred in the 1960s. I would probably have had electric shock treatments or even a lobotomy and would be staring at padded walls now instead of writing this book. At best I would have been a neurotic housewife sipping wine for breakfast and swallowing tranquilizers for dinner.

Humor, I have discovered, is an important part of enjoying life. Therefore I am enjoying this walk down "Memory Lane" to see how far medical science and psychology have advanced in the last quarter century. I was particularly delighted by the following example of an amnesia case of the past. Please note that the evaluation leaves no question as to the cause of the amnesia:

"We begin with an example remarkable for its transparency. A British color-sergeant in World War I was carrying a message, riding his motorcycle through a dangerous section of the front. All at once it was several hours later and he was pushing his motorcycle along the streets of a coastal town nearly a hundred miles away. In utter bewilderment he gave himself up to the military police, but he could tell abolutely nothing of his long trip. The amnesia was ultimately broken by the use of hypnosis. The man then remembered that he was thrown down by a shell explosion, that he picked up himself and his machine, that he started straight for the coastal town, that he studied signs and asked for directions in order to reach his destination.

"It is clear, in this case, that the amnesia entailed no loss of competence. The patient's actions were purposive, rational, and intelligent. The amnesia rested only on his sense of personal identity. The conflict was between fear, suddenly intensified by his narrow escape, and his duty to complete the dangerous mission. The forgetting of personal identity made it possible to give way to his impulse toward flight, now irresistible, without exposing himself to the almost unbearable anxiety associated with being a coward, failing his mission, and undergoing arrest as a deserter. When he achieved physical safety the two sides of the conflict resumed their normal proportions and his sense of personal identity suddenly returned.

"In wartime there are many cases of amnesia and fugue which, like the preceding one, originate under traumatic conditions. In civilian life the same phenomenon occurs under less violent circumstances, but generally in connection with what amounts to an emotional crisis in the patient's life. Some unpleasant social conflict, either financial or familial, was significant in the immediate cause of amnesia, although behind these immediate conflicts deeper motives are found.

"In summary it can be stated that the psychogenic loss of personal identity, such as occurs in amnesias and fugues, represents another way of coping with neurotic conflict. The loss of identity is a defense against intolerable conflict when some powerful need or wish becomes uncontrollable. As is so often true, the wish is ordinarily suppressed because the patient is what he is, occupying a certain social position and having certain responsibilities and obligations. When the wish is so strengthened, usually by some external crisis, that he can no longer keep it suppressed, his personal identity has to be ejected from consciousness."

If all this were true, the hypnosis performed on me should have brought back my past. However, those 48 years are still buried or have been entirely eliminated from my brain. Although there is still the possibility that some of my memory loss is hysterical in nature, doctors seem to agree now that the damage was more physical than psychological. How fortunate I was, then, that the possibility of physical damage was not ruled out as it might have been years ago.

The soldier mentioned in the foregoing anecdote may have suffered a head injury when he was thrown from his motorcycle. He may never have thought of desertion or fear. We will never know. It is amazing to read how simply and categorically the professionals analyzed his problem and solved it.

To cite another, more recent example, after being hit on the head, a man realized that he had had amnesia for 15 years. The accident jarred his memory, and his recollections of a wife and family in another state came flooding back. For 15 years he had lived a quiet life, never remembering his past and never wondering who he had been. As it turned out, he had incurred several blows to the head from accidents and falls, resulting in the lengthy amnesia. I present this case because it is evidence of an amnesia very different from mine and more classic in its symptoms.

As in the case presented from World War I, the patient had no trouble other than being unable to identify who he was and where he had come from. His language and comprehension were unimpaired. However, in this case there was no apparent reason for this lengthy "fugue" state. It did not occur in wartime, and he had no apparent financial or familial problems. As a matter of fact, when he returned to his wife, he found that she was living in the same house and had never remarried because she knew he would return someday. They are presently together and apparently very happy. This casts doubt upon the earlier theory that amnesia is an escape from problems too great for the mind to handle. Of course, we will never know the whole story, but the evidence indicates that the amnesia was induced by a blow to the head and eliminated by a later blow — purely physiological.

The Present

The Neuropsychologist

Although it was exciting to relive the past briefly, it is fascinating to study the advances made since the publication of the aforementioned textbook. I will begin with neuropsychology, an especially interesting and relatively new field. Ten years ago the term "neuropsychology" was unfamiliar. Whereas the psychologist's emphasis is on therapy, the neuropsychologist, with a medical background, emphasizes testing in determining how to treat a patient.

I interviewed several neuropsychologists who are directors of rehabilitation hospitals in the New Jersey-Pennsylvania area, particularly the three psychologists noted in the Bibliography; the facilities in which they practice seem to represent a cross-section of treatment centers. They provided me with a great deal of useful information, which I have combined into the following few pages. Although their techniques vary, there is a vast area of common ground. The neuropsychologist evaluates the brain injured patient to assess the impairment in various areas, e.g., memory, judgment, motivation, and social and emotional behavior. The results of this evaluation are discussed with the family to better understand the effects of the injury. The psychologist should examine the patient shortly after admission and continue the evaluation process regularly throughout the patient's hospitalization. In this way changes can be monitored during recovery.

The Team Approach

At team meetings psychologists discuss their findings with other staff members, and a program of cognitive retraining is formulated. The job of the cognitive retrainer will be discussed later in this chapter, but it should be mentioned here that this job includes aiding the patient in relearning memory and problem solving skills that were lost. The psychologist's role in this process is to help in coordinating the cognitive retraining program so that it is most consistent and effective.

Because a brain injury may affect emotions and behavior, psychotherapy is still another area with which the psychologist must deal. Ideally the patient will develop a close, trusting relationship with the psychologist, and new ways of coping with problems can be explored. Involved in this process is a form of treatment called "behavior modification" in which the patient works with the psychologist to find alternatives to dealing with everyday problems.

The separate jobs of the neuropsychologist, psychologist, and psychiatrist often overlap, although their goals are the same — to help the patient cope with his environment. I have mentioned that the family is often overwhelmed by the stressful results of brain injury, and therefore these professonals must also deal with their problems as well as the patient's. The psychiatrist, with his medical background, can work with others on the team to evaluate the patient and work with the psychology department in decreasing the patient's fears and difficulties in adjusting to his disability.

Doctors often deal with concrete information — CAT scans and electroencephalograms. Neuropsychology is a specialty offering a model of brain-behavior relationships that may be used to relate known, or suspected, brain injuries to observable behavior. In other words, watching and dealing directly with the patient can be more effective than looking at charts and x-ray films. The assessment of this behavior by direct observation is more effective than that achieved by observing structural brain changes after injury. Thus more direct inferences can be made about the limitations in reasoning and performance that will hamper the patient during his daily life.

Working with psychologists and families, the neuropsychologist can help family members recognize the strengths of the "new" family member (the patient), who is learning skills that will help him live more independently.

The Psychologist's Role

I will try to elaborate on the role of psychology in this process of cognitive and social training of the victim of head trauma. Research has shown that many of the interpersonal problems of head injured patients are due to faulty thinking and incorrect assumptions they make about themselves in certain situations. Professionals must deal with the typical childlike quality in adult head injured patients. Sometimes such patients are oversaturated with practicing skills to increase their attention, for example. Even the use of computers, although very helpful (especially at this childlike level), may not help the patient to generalize to other areas of attention and memory.

Fortunately research in this area is progressing systematically to find the answers. Many psychological techniques are being tried in order to improve results. In addition to cognitive deficits, head injured patients have problems in the social-emotional area — impulsivity, lethargy, passivity, catastrophic response to failure, emotional lability, and lowered self-esteem and confidence. The combination of these problems makes it impossible for the patient to function in real-life situations. Consequently many programs of retraining are being implemented using cognitive-social skills and psychological data.

Retraining the Patient

In the early phases of retraining, emphasis is placed on visual attention and concentration. For example, the individuals in a group are told to remember the names of the other group members. Each step is outlined, demonstrated, and reviewed. Group feedback is useful in encouraging this process. At a higher level, techniques of questioning, clarification, and empathy are used.

In later stages the goal is to promote abstract reasoning and problem solving. Again simple exercises such as categorization, analysis of proverbs, and functional problem solving tasks are introduced. Discussion within the group encourages logical thinking and flexibility. One important task is to encourage an understanding of how other people react emotionally to the same situation.

Behavior modification continues with techniques of reinforcement and nonreinforcement (depending on the desired responses), which are adapted as the patient develops less complex skills and goes on to acquire more complex skills. Later neuropsychologists and cognitive retrainers use assertiveness training in handling angry and resistant people and also aid in studying techniques, methods of relaxation, using visual imagery as a memory aid, job interviewing from a psychological aspect, and stress reduction techniques.

The Use of Computers

One tool used in cognitive retraining — computers — is a source of ambivalent feelings among many neuropsychologists and other professionals. Some swear by them as an effective tool in retraining, while others find them useless for all practical purposes.

I would like to present an impartial view of the use of computers in treating head injuries. The reader then can decide for himself.

I have combined information from Barbara Zoltan's book with that gathered from various other professionals in this area to present a fair picture of current attitudes toward computer use for rehabilitative purposes. Chapter 10 of "Perceptual and Cognitive Dysfunction in the Adult Stroke Patient" is solely devoted to "The Use of Computers in Cognitive Retraining." In the next few pages I have included several ideas from that chapter.

In recent years computers have been used in a variety of areas related to head injury — prevocational applications, environmental control, visual, perceptual, or cognitive retraining, and just plain fun. Some professionals believe that computers give head injured patients access to much more of the world than has been possible before. Opponents of computers state that patients must learn to interact with the real world, not with a piece of machinery. Still others state that computers help patients develop fundamental skills needed for everyday activities.

In relation to cognitive retraining, computers can help to increase the capacity for precision, flexibility, and efficiency. Because of immediate and consistent feedback, short presentation times, standardization of training, objectivity, and convenient data storage, patients can benefit from applying skills learned at the computer to other techniques of cognitive retraining.

Many professionals are cautious in their opinion. For example, one states that this retraining may improve eye-hand coordination, attention, and concentration but not the ability to retrieve information from memory. However, one must realize that the object is not to use computers as the only tool of retraining. In conjunction with other techniques, their effectiveness can be enhanced.

I have discovered several possible disadvantages of computers and video games. Early versions of video games, for example, tended to be based on aggressiveness. The availability of software was often limited and sometimes unnecessary for simple retraining. Unfortunately there is little research in the area of computer use in cognitive retraining or other practical activities of daily life, and we must rely on personal opinion at this time.

One study, however, yielded positive results. The objective was to see whether computer retraining was associated with an increase in standardized memory scores and, in turn, whether it had an effect on general memory. The study showed that with time there was in improvement in memory in daily life.

In another case computers were used with head injured patients to increase attention skills, problem solving, visual memory, auditory discrimination, and visual scanning. Patients appeared to be responsive to the program and seemed to progress in the areas of selective attention, improved response time, and increased self-esteem.

Of course these examples are of small selective groups. The results are affected by such outside forces as time, motivation, and family input. Since there is no group to use in comparing results, it is difficult to draw conclusions. Nonetheless there seems to be a strong potential for successful use of computers in the treatment of the head injured. Because there is a great deal of hardware and software available, the therapist must be very selective in choosing what to use. The following are suggested guidelines for this selection obtained by studying available information and interviewing therapists who use this equipment:

1. Games should be simple and uncluttered.
2. Games should require low basic performance levels as well as high ceiling levels.
3. Games should not require much, or any, keyboard input. A joystick, light pen, or space bar should be available for the patient to respond.
4. Use programs that continually adjust to the patient's performance.
5. Use large print letters and numbers.
6. Be aware of the patient's emotional response.
7. Select tools that are simple to use, e.g., cartridges or modules rather than cassettes.

The Selection of Software

Many factors are involved in the intelligent selection of software. The therapist should stay abreast of state of the art software, since new programs are appearing constantly. The therapist should ask the following questions in making these decisions:

1. Is the level of difficulty or complexity of the items controlled and consistent?
2. Can one enter one's own items into the program in addition to using the pre-programed items?
3. Are instructions concise and easy to follow?
4. Is the response format consistent so that the learner does not become confused?
5. Is the content accurate? Are any parts of the program demeaning?
6. How much supervision, if any, is needed in order for the patient to run the program?
7. What type of feedback is supplied to the user?
8. What variables can one control (e.g., the length of time the stimulus is displayed, the time that elapses until the patient must respond, the level of difficulty, the speed of task performance, the size of the letters, and the time and type of reinforcement)?
9. How are errors represented?
10. How are data kept and reported?
11. Does the program provide instructions on the screen?

These guidelines and questions apply to all decisions dealing with the use of the computer as a retraining tool. Even those opposed to its use in cognitive retraining find it a source of entertainment and some skill development. Nonetheless a decision about the use of computers depends ultimately on financial considerations. More research with positive results will have to be done before many facilities will support the outlay of large sums of money to provide computers and software for head injured patients.

Cognitive Retraining

With or without computers, the job of the cognitive retrainer often overlaps the roles of the neuropsychologist, psychologist, and psychiatrist. Using a daily journal, taking notes, and using different sensory modalities and repetitious memory task training are a few of the techniques that can be systematically taught. Cognitive retraining is often a long and tedious process, but it is well worth the effort. To recapitulate briefly what we already have learned in various chapters of this book, the major focus of the cognitive retrainer is on six specific areas, as delineated in "The Head Trauma Family Guide" printed for Lourdes Regional Rehabilitation Center in Camden, NJ:

1. Arousal, attention, and concentration. In order to learn anything, a patient must first be able to pay attention. To maintain concentration, highly structured, focused exercises are employed.

2. Memory. Memory is important in everyday functioning. There are various degrees and kinds of memory loss, and each must be dealt with on an individual basis with specific exercises to improve memory.

3. Sequencing. Some patients cannot plan their actions or carry them out in the correct order. Such "simple" activities as dressing and eating have to be dealt with.

4. Abstract-verbal skills. In most social situations the patient needs to use language and abstract thinking. Here there is often difficulty in vocabulary, poor categorization skills (seeing similarities and differences between objects), and concrete thinking (seeing the point of view of others, for example). Thinking in abstract terms is a major consideration in treatment.

5. Visual-motor skills. Some skills are more visual and nonverbal. These include everyday mechanical tasks and having a general sense of direction.

6. Social-emotional skills. Here are included all the subtle skills needed in everyday social situations — carrying on approprate conversation, being aware of one's own and others' feelings, and having a sense of humor. They also include reducing impulsiveness and increasing confidence and self-esteem as well as dealing with the patient's sexual concerns.

To explain how therapists go about evaluating these areas of cognitive deficit, the foregoing has been broken down into specific categories:

Attention

The word "attention" describes many kinds of behavior. It is defined as "a function which ensures that cognitive processing is directed towards the significant features of the environment . . . a state of arousal allowing the individual to receive information and attend to it; contains the three components of alertness, selectivity, and effort." Attention is a process that determines what is important to the individual. Alertness is just a part of attention. It is related to preparing the patient to be attentive. Concentration, vigilance, and effort involve the ability to sustain attention over a period of time.

There are two types of information processing that are related to attention — automatic and controlled processing. When new information is being considered, controlled processing is utilized. The automatic processing occurs at a subcortical level, using previously acquired information.[1] Several tests are used to determine the extent of attention impairment.

Random Letter Test

The evaluator reads a long list of random letters and asks the patient to somehow indicate when he hears a predetermined letter. Letters are read at the rate of one per second. The scoring is nonstandardized. The patient should complete the test without any errors. To make this test more effective, hearing and language deficits must first be ruled out as a cause of poor performance.

Digit Repetition Test

The evaluator states random number sequences and asks the patient to say the same numbers after she is finished. Here again, numbers are presented at a rate of one per second. The scoring is also nonstandardized. A patient with average intelligence should be able to repeat five to seven digits. Less than five indicates defective attention.

Clinical Observation and Activity Analysis

Here the evaluator must identify the components of attention that are intact and those that are impaired, observe the patient in various settings and activities, and establish functional baseline measures by selecting relevant tasks for the evaluation.

After these tests have been given and all aspects of the patient's condition have been examined, the next step is treatment to improve attention. Because environment can affect performance, training must begin in a nondistracting environment in a structured manner. As improvement occurs, the structure is decreased and the patient is introduced to a more normal environment. During this period there should be feedback to modify behavior and rewards for increased attention to a task. The length of treatment can be increased as the patient progresses. External cues should be provided to help the patient increase his awareness of his surroundings. Internal attentional strategies, such as asking the patient to say what he is going to do, step by step, will help train him to think about what he will do.

Controlled sensory cuing is the next stage in treatment. The patient is given a sensory cue (visual, tactile, or auditory), and then he must perform a particular task. Once he grasps simple ideas, the tasks become more complex. One hopes that learning in one area will affect learning in similar areas. For example, a patient who has learned to recognize numbers can learn to identify colored numbers by their color.[1]

At this point many therapists recommend the use of computers with programs specifically designed to remedy attentional deficits, in conjunction with all, or at least several, of the other techniques described.

Memory

Memory is perception that has been stored at an earlier time and then can be brought forward.[1] There are several types of memory:

1. Recognition: part of recall; a primitive function that alerts the patient to his surroundings.

2. Iconic: sensory memory.

3. Short term: lasts only 20 to 40 seconds (for example, memorizing five or 10 items immediately after they are heard).

4. Long term: represents a permanent record of learned material. This is composed of three stages — consolidation, storage, and retrieval (recall).[1]

To evaluate memory, the therapist must try to separate it from other cognitive functions. The standardized tests available often are not specific enough to determine memory deficit alone. It is helpful, then, to include family reports and patient reports. The most effective tests include the following:

Wechsler Memory Scale

This scale includes personal and current information, orientation, mental control, logical memory, digit span, visual reproduction, and associative learning. The scoring tests short term memory digit span, associative verbal memory, meaningful verbal memory, and figural memory in a standardized fashion.

Subjective Memory Questionnaire

This questionnaire includes 43 items relating to everyday life, such as names, facts about people, and film titles. The answers are scored on a five point rating scale from "very good" to "very bad" and from "very rarely" to "very often."

Clinical Observation and Activity Analysis

As in analyzing attention deficits, the therapist's evaluation from observation is most important in identifying memory deficits. The treatment for these deficits includes maintaining a consistent routine and environment; controlling the environment; providing a little training more frequently rather than too much for too long; and using memory aids such as rehearsal, elaborating, compatibility, visual imagery, mnemonics (letters and rhymes that cue the patient); as well as external aids like alarm clocks, diaries, labeling, writing notes, or providing verbal or visual cues.[1]

Initiation

Initiation refers to the ability to start something or respond without instructions to do so. A patient with no initiative, apathy, and general lethargy exhibits characteristics of a deficit in initiation. The only way to evaluate such a problem at this time is through direct clinical observation and activity analysis. There are no standardized or nonstandardized tests to measure this problem.

The treatment of initiation deficits is quite basic — continual repetition and cuing are provided until the patient gradually improves and is able to cue himeself internally. Sensory input is useful along with auditory cuing.[1]

Sequencing

Closely related to initiation are the areas of "planning and organization" as well as "sequencing." In order to formulate a goal, the patient must be able to define what he needs and wants to achieve that goal. Certain steps must be taken mentally to come up with a plan, and these steps must be carried out in proper order for the goal to be achieved. Involved in this process are the abilities to foresee change and to think logically.

As in the areas of deficiency mentioned previously, testing can be done only by direct observation. By asking a patient what he intends to do, a therapist can quickly judge whether there is a defect in his planning skills. If there is more than one step in a particular task, the patient's deficits will quickly be evidenced by his inability to perform the given task.

To treat these planning and organization deficits, the therapist must control the amount and time of feedback. She can help by providing planning aids (e.g., written step by step instructions). Eventually the goal is to have the patient use internal questioning techniques like asking himself, "What is it I want to accomplish?" The patient then can write down a plan and try to achieve it. Simple tasks will lead, ideally, to more complex tasks, and the need for external cuing will decrease.[1]

Mental Flexibility and Abstraction Deficits

Mental flexibility and abstraction (or abstract-verbal skills) deficits are signaled by difficulty in learning new information or in using old information properly. When there is poor mental flexibility, the patient often perseverates (constantly repeats). In other words he cannot generalize to solve future problems. He is stuck in a limbo filled with useless information.

To evaluate mental flexibility, there a test called "Odd-Even Cross-out." The patient is given a worksheet with a series of numbers on it. He is asked to cross out all the even numbers at first, and then partially through he is to switch to crossing out the odd numbers. The directions change back and forth several times until the test is completed. The results effectively demonstrate the patient's mental flexibility and the degree to which it has been impaired.

To evaluate abstraction, a test consists of concept formation and abstraction. Sample questions include the following:

1. Definition-abstraction: The patient is asked to define a specific word.

2. Comparison-differentiation: The patient is asked to relate a pair of ideas through common ground and differences.

3. Logical relationships: The patient is asked to relate a word to a given series.

4. Opposites: The patient is asked to supply the opposite of a word.

5. Categories: The patient is asked to identify the word that does not belong in a series of words.

6. Proverbs: The patient is asked to give the meanings of a series of proverbs.

Results from these tests clearly show difficulty in abstraction. To treat this problem, the therapist uses a functional approach by asking the patient to perform various tasks in addition to using computers to improve performance. Repetition, again, is the most useful tool.[1]

In the area of social-emotional skills, we find the subjects of "decreased insight and impulsivity." Many patients deny that there is any problem at all. Because he does not recognize his limitations, the patient may be impulsive and rash in his behavior. Some patients can recognize their limitations but cannot do anything about their behavior. For example, a patient who is paralyzed and who cannot control his own behavior may fall out of bed in trying to walk.

This deficit can be recognized only through observation. Treatment must be given in a nondistracting environment, providing close monitoring and feedback, including discussion, observation, demonstration, and repetition. Tasks are provided that gradually demonstrate deficits as well as the patient's strengths. This initially may cause depression, which can be overcome with patience, understanding, and eventual acceptance by the patient. Finally, verbal and tactile cuing is used in conjunction with other techniques to "remind" the patient of his limitations.

Problem Solving

Combining several categories mentioned already, patients often suffer from a deficiency in the area of problem solving. Here are combined the skills of attention, memory, organization, planning, and judgment. Difficulty with any of these skills will affect problem solving. The process of problem solving itself can be summarized as follows:

1. Begin with a problem.

2. Formulate it in an active and dynamic cognitive act within the particular context in which it occurs.

3. Analyze the conditions of the problem that are most pertinent, in the given context, to a solution.

4. When the analysis is completed and the salient features of the problem have been identified by the patient, the next phase in the process begins — choosing an approach to the solution from several alternatives.

5. Once a strategy has been decided upon, the patient must formulate a working plan, which involves setting priorities, selecting sequences of action, determining the tactics to be employed, and careful correlating of these so that they make up a coherent working plan.

6. Following completion of this process, the patient begins to execute the plan.

7. This in turn requires constant monitoring of one's behavior and verifying that each step is being executed according to the original plan of action.

8. If all goes well, the patient then arrives at a solution to the problem.

9. He must then compare the solution obtained with that defined in the original problem.

10. Once the solution is found to be acceptable, the patient performs an explicit or implicit mental act of evaluating the significance of the achievement. This cognitive process culminates in the integration of the achievement with the patient's other relevant goals and behavior patterns.[1]

In one test used to determine whether there is a deficit in problem solving the patient is asked to reproduce a block design constructed by the examiner. While the patient is doing this the examiner records his progress. A deficit is evident if the patient seems disorganized or is unable to compare.

More subjective testing involves observation by the therapist. It is easier to identify a difficulty in problem solving than to treat the difficulty. Many previously mentioned techniques of monitoring, providing external cues, and repetition along with computers, log books, and verbal cues can systematically work to improve the patient's problem solving abilities.

The techniques just described apply to both head injured patients and stroke patients. Positive results help to reinforce the theory that cognitive retraining is effective in helping the patient toward living a useful life. I must warn the reader, however, that these techniques do not always work. Sometimes the injury is too severe, and no technique is effective. However, not until we have tried every available method can we give up hope.

Nonetheless we must realize that there will be cases that are beyond help. In those cases the family must decide when to stop.[1]

The Nurse

One profession that should be mentioned here is one that is invaluable in the treatment and recovery of head injured patients — nursing. All of the source material from the various hospitals and rehabilitation centers shared the same opinion of the importance of this vital branch of the team. Beginning with the intensive care (or trauma) nurse, through the primary registered nurse to the practical nurse and the rehabilitation nurse, all members of this profession serve a vital role in the care of patients.

In other chapters I have given credit to the nurses who carry out the daily routine responsibilities in the patient's care. However, here I would like to mention the rehabilitation nurse, who works in conjunction with the therapist and neuropsychologist. Her job varies according to the conditions of the patient. If his physical condition is very serious, she is responsible for evaluating the daily needs in relation to positioning, bowel and bladder functioning, hygiene, physical health, and neurological status.

The rehabilitation nurse consults daily with the attending physicians in regard to the patient's progress so that treatment can be modified as changes occur. As the patient improves, the nurse provides bladder and bowel training and assists in the retraining of self-care skills. In many cases these nurses work for insurance companies or private agencies to coordinate the patient's rehabilitation.

The Facilitator

Everything I have discussed since the beginning of Chapter 7 has involved the professionals who deal with the patient and his family in a hospital or rehabilitation setting. What happens when the patient is sent home? Many continue to return to the rehabilitation center for outpatient treatment. However, recently a relatively new occupation has arisen out of a demand for home care and continued therapy on an intensive level, that of the "facilitator." Crossroads Healthcare Services, Inc. of Jenkintown, Pennsylvania, an organization which employs and utilizes such facilitators, provided much of the following information concerning their job. The facilitator is responsible for the "implementation of the client's treatment plan in accordance with the goals and objectives formulated by the rehabilitation team," which may include:

1. Systematic application of therapeutic regimens outlined by the various disciplines (such as speech and language, physiotherapy, occupational therapy, cognitive remediation, behavior modification, and psychology).

2. Planning and implementing training in daily living skills, personal hygiene, grooming, clothing care, and household maintenance, in addition to supervising and monitoring the patient's execution of these tasks.

3. In coordination with the therapeutic team, planning, implementing, supervising, and instructing the patient in social and recreational activities (including transportation to these activities or training him in utilizing transportation services to community based activities as appropriate).

4. Assisting the family in learning specific techniques related to the patient's treatment regimen and personal care and safety in the community.

5. Serving as a member of the rehabilition team by participating in the implementation of the patient's rehabilitation treatment on a continuing basis, by consulting with members of the team, the family, and other professionals in order to plan, implement, and evaluate the treatment plan, and by communicating to the therapeutic staff the potential effectiveness or the necessity for adopting or restructuring specific program objectives.

6. Completing daily progress notes and other reports as required.

The facilitator is thus a jack of all trades. She employs all the techniques of the various disciplines in the home environment and in daily activities. Although different therapists may come throughout the week, the facilitator is there every day, often for eight to 12 hours at a time. Because she is there so frequently, she must also work with the family, helping them adjust to the patient's limitations. She is thus a therapist, counselor, advisor, and friend. This is a great deal to ask of one person, but the facilitators whom I interviewed regard it as very rewarding work.

Sometimes eight hours a day with one person is too much. In such a case perhaps two facilitators can take four-hour shifts each day to provide variety and stimulation for the patient. These two would work as a team, reinforcing each other's efforts and thus provide consistency for the patient.

The facilitator is a resource person who helps the therapists working with the patient. Most organizations that provide facilitators for home care have certain requirements concerning education and experience. For example, they may require an advanced degree in rehabilitation, psychology, sociology, social work, or special education, or perhaps a bachelor's degree will suffice with certain levels of experience, or even an associate degree with more experience in the health care field.

There are many more important considerations. Common sense, self control, and consistency weigh more heavily than a diploma. This job is very demanding and emotionally draining. In the home setting the facilitator must deal constantly with the patient and the family, and the relationship has to be a positive one in order for progress to occur.

Certain skills are required before one begins to work with a brain injured patient. The facilitator must have a knowledge of brain injuries, their treatment, and their social implications. She must also have some knowledge of medications, their proper dosages, and expected results, since most head injured patients require such treatment. It is also helpful if she is familiar with teaching and training techniques as well as techniques of behavior modification.

Aside from knowledge and skills, the facilitator must be endowed with the abilities to follow through on the details of program planning, to understand and follow oral and written instructions of a technical nature, to maintain a positive attitude, to recognize and identify patient problems and make emergency decisions, to prepare and maintain a variety of forms and records, and to establish and maintain effective working relationships with patients, their families, staff members, and other professionals in the field.

The work of the facilitator goes far beyond a typical "job description." It is unfortunate that such a job did not exist when I was injured. I did have a nurse at home for a while, but she was more of a baby-sitter than a therapist. I am hoping that more training programs will be provided throughout the country to increase the availability of these facilitators and, particularly, that insurance companies will be more responsive to the demand for such care.

The Social Worker and Other Sources of Help for the Patient

There are many people, not in the medical fields, whose services are invaluable to the victim of head trauma. For example, the social worker, employed by the hospital or a social service agency (such as the welfare department), acts as a liaison between the professional team and others concerned with the patient, including family, funding sources, friends, and past or future employers. She is often the source of information or direction for distraught families. The information she compiles about the patient also will be useful for later treatment, particularly orientation and memory deficits.

Although the social worker is not directly involved with the patient's treatment, without her assessment (including the patient's history, pretrauma personality style, educational history, developmental milestones, leisure interests, skills, and family input), the professional treatment staff would have a more difficult time setting rehabilitation goals or making long range plans.

In recent years more emphasis has been placed on the needs and interests of head injured patients by many others outside the medical profession, for example, insurance companies as well as attorneys who are fighting to protect patients' legal rights. Partly because it is so widespread, head injury is becoming a very specialized field. This development can only lead to greater advances in research, treatment, and public concern.

In the remaining chapters I will attempt to evaluate our present approach to treatment and suggest how we can learn from each other in order to improve what we now have. My goal is to educate, or at least to open a few eyes to an important topic. If one person will benefit from my words, then I have succeeded.

References

1. Siev E, Freishtat B, Zoltan B: Perceptual and Cognitive Dysfunction in the Adult Stroke Patient. Thorofare, NJ: Slack, Inc., 1986, pp. 110-133.

11

What Have We Learned?

Drawing conclusions from a set of facts and opinions is a very subjective task, and one can read the preceding chapters and reject or accept whatever one chooses. I have attempted to present the information in this book from the viewpoints of everyone involved with head trauma — the families, the professionals, and the victims themselves. My own experience of course introduces some bias but, it is hoped, only in the direction of improving the current techniques and treatment used in rehabilitation.

Six years of observation and personal involvement as well as almost a year of intensive research (interviewing, attending seminars and workshops, and visiting rehabilitation facilities throughout Pennsylvania and New Jersey) have led me to develop strong feelings about what has been done, what is presently being done, and what needs to be done. The last question is dealt with in the Epilogue. Here I shall use the preceding information to draw conclusions and give an overview of the present situation.

The National Head Injury Foundation, headquartered in Framingham, Massachusetts, has formulated a list of their major goals. I am presenting them here because they also represent some of my goals in writing this book.

Goal: Increase public, family, and professional awareness of the silent epidemic.

Objectives:

A. Publish and distribute newsletters, brochures, and informational pamphlets.

B. Undertake a national awareness media campaign.

C. Hold educational seminars for both families and professionals, and participate in national conferences committed to treatment and prevention.

Goal: Lobby to achieve recognition of the problem of head injury and the needs of those who have suffered head injuries.

Objectives:

A. Make direct presentations of the problem to federal and state agencies and to the insurance industry.

B. Create special task forces to define the funding and treatment needs of those who have sustained head injuries.

C. Keep membership aware of legislative matters of concern to the head injured population and stimulate legislative action.

Goal: Create an information and resource center for head injury.

Objectives:

A. Establish a national "help line."

B. Disseminate resource information in the NHIF newsletter.

C. Publish a complete listing of head injury rehabilitation facilities.

D. Assist chapters in compiling local resource directories.

E. Develop comprehensive head injury resource library.

Goal: Develop a unifying structure to provide support for the survivors of head injury and their families.

Objectives:

A. Expand the NHIF national membership base, including those who have suffered head injuries, their families and friends, and professionals.

B. Establish NHIF chapters throughout the country and develop family support groups within chapters.

Goal: Assist in the establishment of rehabilitation programs for the head injured population - from coma to community.

Objectives:

A. Identify "models of care" from acute injury to late rehabilitation.

B. Develop guidelines for late rehabilitation programs with emphasis on cognitive remediation, family support, independent living skills, and vocational retraining.

C. Undertake national fund-raising to provide seed money for program development.

Goal: Raise monies to support research.

Objectives:

A. Support basic research on the mechanism and repair of central nervous function.

B. Support innovative techniques and programs in head injury rehabilitation at all levels.

Goal: Prevention.

Objectives:

Support activities and legislation related to accident prevention and highway safety aimed at reducing head injuries and fatalities.

The goal of prevention is a vast area of concern. Presently we are seeing television documentaries on drunk driving and seat belt use. These are quite effective, but need to be seen by more viewers. A simple solution to that problem would be to require these films to be shown at school assemblies. Legislation is being proposed to enforce seat belt use nationally, provide stricter enforcement of drunk driving penalties, and determine the responsibility of those serving alocholic beverages to potential drivers.

Statistics suggest that stricter enforcement leads to fewer accidents. Although the public may be outraged by what seems to be an infringement of its rights, take a look at "Nick" sitting awkwardly in his wheelchair, unable to feed himself or carry on a conversation, and compare that to the outrage!

We victims of head trauma are very special people. Although our individual differences are vast, there is a common bond. The existence of this bond makes it necessary for the head injured to be around each other, to realize that they are not alone. Unfortunately, some victims of head trauma are placed in rehabilitation centers filled primarily with stroke victims and amputees. There are also some facilities without neuropsychologists or family counselors.

This is not always the case, however. There are several wonderful centers that are very progressive and family oriented. Unfortunately there are not as any as needed. Where do we place a victim of head trauma who has progressed as far as he can through rehabilitation but still cannot function independently? I have known of spouses and children suffering for periods of 12 or 13 years while searching for a suitable facility. Many nursing homes are not equipped to satisfy the needs of such victims. Their staff members are totally unfamiliar, for the most part, with head trauma, and the care is unstructured and unsuitable for the needs of the head injured.

The care given today in the majority of nursing homes is designed for the aged, the senile, and the sickly. Death appears to be the only ultimate alternative. Where in this setting is there a place for Nick (discussed in Chapter 3), who is in his 20's and needs around the clock care? Is there also a place for him to live a useful and happy life?

The more I talk with families, victims, and professionals, the more I recognize what is missing. Although I have found many dedicated and selfless professionals, they are all hampered by "the system." Money is an important factor that cannot be discounted. Many rehabilitation facilities have high ideals and competent staffs, but they are shackled by the restraints imposed by the budget. The only reasonable solution in these cases is the proper allotment of available funds. Many techniques now being used are outdated and ineffective. One psychologist, the director of a nearby outpatient care department within a rehabilitation center, commented that he would rather have the money spent on kitchen equipment (to teach the patients practical techniques in self-care and living) than on a shipment of computers. Let me emphasize that he was not downgrading the usefulness of computers. They have proved very effective in occupational therapy (in training a patient for a computer related job or for teaching games for the patient to play with others). However, looking at the total picture, one wonders how useful a computer can be when the patient cannot make himself a sandwich.

This example undoubtedly will spur a heated debate, but that is a positive reaction. At least it will bring the issue to public notice, and perhaps a compromise can be achieved. In another case, when rehabilitation techniques have proved fruitless and the patient is merely existing, what should be done? I have met several patients who always sleep through therapy and have shown no improvement in years. Considering the financial as well as emotional drain on the families, could the money to finance such therapy be put to better use - perhaps in providing a total-care facility where the family can visit in addition to taking the patient out for regular excursions or home visits? Professionals need to work more with families to make such decisions.

Another important aspect of head trauma is the law. I am most familiar with what is happening in New Jersey, but the situation here is indicative of the changes occurring around the country. We are in effect a test case for other states in regard to legal dealings with head injury. At present victims and families have a good chance of being free of many financial worries, because there are no limitations on awards for "pain, suffering, and permanent damage" due to catastrophic illness. This benefits everyone (except for the insurance companies); help is provided for a lifetime if the injury is permanent. With all the problems associated with head injury, it is a relief to know that at least the family's financial worries are over.

However, legislation is now pending to put a $300,000 limit on such payment. That meager amount, in comparison to rehabilitation costs and medical expenses, is but a drop in the bucket! Amazingly, statistics show that that insurance companies made a national profit this year of over $8 billion! Stock brokers recommend investing in insurance companies because of their financial potential. Nonetheless, these very companies now say that they are losing money and wish to reduce benefits. Because of the lobbying power of these companies, new legislation is steadily eating away at the rights of victims an their families.

I am overwhelmed by this subject. I cannot understand how a lovely lady I met has lost her home and is barely subsisting after 13 years of caring for her head injured husband. They are receiving too much money to be eligible for public assistance, yet not enough to survive.

Currently New Jersey's minimum mandatory auto liability policy is for $15,000. In the treatment of head injury, that would barely cover a brief hospital stay, and would not begin to act as compensation for pain and suffering.

Other legal issues include questions of guardianship, symptoms occurring long after an injury, and insurance settlements. I can only recommend that families seek competent legal representation with someone very familiar with head injury cases. This is an area that is relatively new and untested, so the search for representation may be a difficult one.

In the long run, however, individuals cannot change the legal situation on their own. The chances of improving benefits seem small due to the overwhelming power of those opposed to the idea. Clearly, the only possible solution is public opinion. One voice is but a fleeting puff of smoke; many voices can produce a storm!

As seen in Chapter 3, every case is different. There are varying degrees of long term and short term memory loss, physical limitation, and progress. Therefore there can be no uniform treatment during rehabilitation. It follows, then, that programs of rehabilitation must be flexible. The training of therapists must extend further than a semester course in rehabilitation training.

My visit to one rehabilitation center, in particular, was enlightening. Staff members were very cooperative in providing information and answering my questions. When asked what the major problem was for the victims and their families, the director's immediate response was "acceptance." Being a psychologist, he was able to go more deeply into the complex ramifications of the word. "Acceptance" is defined as "receiving willingly." This is far different from "coping," which is "struggling or contending, perhaps successfully." I have found that coping is usually the appropriate word when it comes to dealing with head trauma. Acceptance seems to imply a giving up, when in actuality it implies showing strength. The patient and his family can find satisfaction in learning to accept the limitations imposed by the injury and work to the maximum of his ability. Too often patients and their families live in the past. One hears a parent or spouse say, "I can't forget what he used to be like." People often cling to a dream that one day the patient will wake up and be the same as he was before the accident. This dream makes acceptance impossible.

A common goal of the victim of head trauma is to go back to his old job. Often this cannot happen, and so he must be retrained, if possible, for a job that he can handle successfully. In a hypothetical case a patient suffers head trauma and is then rehabilitated to the point at which he can go back to work. Perhaps he is not doing as complex a job as he once did, but he is, nevertheless, working. When a problem arises that would be considered "typical" (a personality conflict with a coworker or a complaint by a customer, for example), the victim's response may be blown out of proportion. He is often treated as "sick" because of his past experience. Had the same experience happened to anyone else, the response might very well be the same without its being considered unusual. Likewise in a young patient, normal teenage behavior may be considered mistakenly to be a result of the head injury. Parents may allow unacceptable behavior because they do not understand that the behavior is typical of the normal teenager.

When these reactions are thought to be pathological, it is time for information, not psychotherapy. The patient needs guidance and facts to understand what is happening to him. Typical life is like a graph, with many ups and downs. Following head trauma the level goes down, far below the previous lowest level. When stability returns to the patient's life, the degree of the low is intensified when a problem arises, often with depression or an overreaction.

Particularly when the victim is the child, many families have trouble "letting go." The normal separation of parent and child is difficult enough. After head trauma, when the parent or spouse becomes the nurse and teacher as well as protector of the victim, it is even more difficult to allow the child to grow and gain independence. It is a natural instinct to want to protect, even when it is no longer in the best interests of the patient. Family members may feel threatened or useless if they are no longer "needed."

This is the time for family guidance. Unfortunately present-day coverage by insurance companies rarely allows compensation for family counseling. Most families cannot afford this much needed therapy. The only alternative, which is just now gaining in popularity, is the self-help support groups. In time such groups will be available on a large scale, but they do not fill all the needs of the family.

In one rehabilitation center I recently visited, I was pleased to see concern for the needs of the patient as well as those of the family. Because it is an outpatient center, the therapy is aimed at preparing the patient for life on the outside. Usually this means training in self-help skills, shopping, budgeting, cooking, or making beds. In other cases the patient can be retrained for a job. Help is given in learning specific tasks, interviewing techniques, and general work routines. In all cases goals are set. As time passes, expectations sometimes are lowered to lessen frustration when progress is slow.

After a child goes to school for many years, he graduates and goes to find a job, realizing that he has learned little practical information related directly to his work. Likewise, vocational rehabilitation may have little to do with the patient's future job. Therefore many rehabilitation centers are training patients for specific jobs. For example, a prospective secretary was trained using the same typewriter and adding machine that she would have on the job. She was able to achieve a higher level of proficiency at work because of this extensive training.

It is not difficult to identify the problems that patients and their families have to face in dealing with head trauma. The question is, How effective are present-day therapies? The answers are debatable. While searching for information for Chapters 7 to 10 I came to some conclusions about these matters.

To begin with, as in all professions, there are all types of therapists. The quality and dedication depend on the individual as well as the institution for which he works. Occupational therapy is a profession that demands a high degree of dedication. Few centers can afford to pay what the therapist is really worth, yet the jobs are filled. Frequently therapists have to make the best of what are perhaps scant resources or inadequate facilities.

Working with the victims of head trauma can often be frustrating and depressing. One must detach oneself emotionally or suffer through the pain of each patient. On the other hand, the satisfaction and sense of accomplishment gained from working with victims of head trauma make all the struggle worthwhile. To see a response in a comatose patient for whom doctors held little hope or to see a previously useless limb start to function is a reward whose value is beyond calculation.

Many conclusions drawn from the preceding information would seem to be obvious. However, the very people from whom the information was collected are often surprised that their feelings and experiences are so common. Each person believes his experience is unique. For example, my lengthy amnesia seemed to have no similarity to Mary's short-term difficulties. However, upon deeper investigation I can see how we are alike. What appears obvious to the outsider is often unrecognizable to those in the midst of the turmoil created by head injury.

For example, here I am speaking out publicly, able to drive a car, run a household, and function each day by myself. What people cannot see is where I was six years ago. They cannot see the hysteria, the confusion, the vulgarity, or the inability to function on my own.

Even though my memory loss is long term, I still have to keep accurate account of everything I do. I write notes everywhere. I keep a notebook with me at all times to remind me of things I would otherwise forget. Sometimes I revert to the child within me, the child I was immediately following my accident. It is an escape from the confusion and frustration of living in such an anxiety filled world. Perhaps I am more fortunate than most: I can choose who I want to be to suit the occasion. People seem to be in awe of what I have accomplished, yet I feel lacking in many areas. I would like to have a more proficient vocabulary; I would like to remember things without writing them down. Sometimes the little girl in me remembers feeling "stupid," and it is a difficult feeling to forget.

I realize how fortunate I am. I only wish that all the other victims of head trauma can have the opportunity to progress as far as possible. No one is able to cure the ills of the world, but we all can succeed in making life more enjoyable and more productive for those who inhabit it.

12

Epilogue
What's Next?

This last chapter is the culmination of years of experience and hours of interviewing. I do not profess to be an expert on head injury or to suggest that my beliefs represent the only solutions to problems associated with head trauma. However, I do want to present an alternative, a possible way of dealing with a serious and confusing situation. I will be the first to admit that there is no single simple solution to everyone's problems; in some cases there may be no solution. The best that can be hoped for is the ability to cope with an unbearable situation.

Throughout medical history there has been a reluctance to explore the unexplored. Breakthroughs are long in coming because of fear. New techniques, especially in medicine, are tested innumerable times, and even then there is a reluctance to accept positive results. In dealing with head trauma, however, there is hope that new or refined methods of treatment can be combined with tried-and-true techniques in an effort to totally rehabilitate the patient.

The following suggestions are presented in no particular order of importance, for the treatment depends largely on the severity of the injuries and the head trauma.

1. Therapy during coma. The need for this cannot be minimized. Patients in coma do respond to outside stimuli; the more stimuli, the better the chance of arousal to a conscious state. I have mentioned touching, massaging, talking, and playing favorite music. I would also include moving the patient, if possible. Take him outdoors in a wheelchair. Sounds, smells, temperature changes, and tactile stimulation are useful tools. Physical therapy during coma keeps the body toned and helps to prevent atrophy, foot drop, pressure sores, and spasms.

Speech pathologists are now realizing the effectiveness of using headsets with the patient who is in a coma to eliminate outside noise, which can be distracting. Often the sounds we want the patient to hear, the music and the familiar voices, are drowned out by the normal sounds of a hospital. By using headsets, the sounds we want the patient to hear are separated and directed to the patient. This technique has proved successful in that we can now recognize the patient's reaction to the sounds — increased heart rate and respiration, and flexibility of the ear drum, or tympanic membrance. Although the patient may not understand what he hears, he is indeed listening.

2. Family involvement in therapy. If there are family members nearby who can help, the progress of rehabilitation will be enhanced. Repetition works as well as determination. The patient must realize that he is not alone. Even when there is no family, the staff can provide needed psychological support, particularly social workers and counselors.

In every rehabilitation center I visited, family involvement was the norm. In times of great stress human beings tend to rally around those who need help. Of course there are those who have no families or whose families have abandoned them. The patients involved in the research for this book were fortunate to have this important support group.

3. Dealing with the patient at his learning developmental level. It must first be determined how old the patient is developmentally. Then the therapists, doctors, and family members can relate to the patient at his own level, remembering that he may quickly grow beyond this age and need to be treated accordingly. Therapists in particular must show the patient what is to be done, not just tell him. Verbal cues should be used to stimulate physical action. Repetition, again, reinforces the learning of skills, and praise helps the patient feel a sense of accomplishment in completing the smallest task.

4. Rewards. In the beginning, especially when the patient's learning developmental age is quite young, simple rewards are conducive to learning. Later these rewards are more often verbal or physical. A hug can mean as much as a toy. Eventually the patient may find his own reward in his sense of accomplishment and pride.

5. Letting the patient be the teacher. Once a skill has been mastered, there is no greater reward for the patient than to teach another patient how to perform that skill. Many who have gone through every available therapy and still cannot find a job would be overjoyed at the opportunity to show other victims of head trauma what they can do. Teaching is an area that they can perform well in and feel comfortable with because they know what other similar patients are going through. It is conceivable that rehabilitation centers could hire rehabilitated victims of head trauma to work with their present patients.

6. Combining counseling with all other forms of rehabilitation. Repairing the body alone is useless without repairing the mind. These therapies must be used together to integrate the patient back into society. When there is little hope of the patient's recovering enough to live independently, he and his family will need help in adjusting to his limitations. Even when the patient can return to a relatively normal life, he may need counseling to accept the fact that there are some differences he must live with. It seems

that almost everyone in the 1980s faces more stress than ever before. The added problem of head trauma creates a necessity to seek outside help in dealing with these additional pressures.

7. Developing rehabilitation programs that work together with the families and employing the aforementioned techniques to treat the patient. More and more rehabilitation centers are developing separate head trauma departments, but the expansion is not catching up to the demand for more facilities. Head trauma is a nationwide epidemic that needs federal involvement. Certain diseases have foundations whose spokesmen are national celebrities even though that disease affects only a small percentage of the population. With head trauma we have a "silent epidemic" that is relatively unheard of and in desperate need of public exposure.

8. Encouraging the use of successful techniques not yet in widespread use. A relatively new technique, best known in the Southeast, is now catching on throughout the country — biofeedback or electromyography (the recording of electrical impulses from muscles). Though not a miracle cure for restoring lost function, it has helped hundreds of patients recover some portion of their lost abilities after other techniques had failed. Biofeedback is combined with physical therapy to improve movement, coordination, and activities for daily living. A 1975 publication by the Biofeedback Research Institute provided much of the following information.[1]

Biofeedback has been in use for approximately 50 years as a diagnostic and prognostic procedure for determining state of an individual's muscles and nerves and making predictions about recovery. The original machinery used to record these impulses was a large, expensive electromyograph (EMG). Today, however, small, portable, battery-operated versions (called electromyometers or EMMs) have been designed in conjunction with computers.

Although the technique is more than half a century old, it was not until the 1950s and that the use of the EMG as a therapeutic tool began to be studied. Dr. Alberto Marinacci and Dr. J. G. Golseth were pioneers in the clinical application of biofeedback in neuromuscular reeducation.

It was discovered at that time that the patients having the best possibility of recovery were those with a considerable amount of latent function present. For example, I have a friend who can cross her right little toe over the toe next to it. By concentrating very hard, she can control the muscle in her toe. However, when she tries the same thing with her left toe nothing happens. The left toe muscle is evident to the touch, so there is no obvious latent function present.

Similarly, muscles that have not been entirely destroyed have the potential for retraining. In the 50s little was known about head trauma, so this use for biofeedback was unknown. They did know, however, that there was a considerable amount of potential for recovery in stroke patients (often considered similar to head injury patients in symptoms and treatment).

The methods suggested in the 1950s were not commonly used until recently because articles about biofeeedback were published in little-read journals. Not until smaller, less expensive instruments were designed was there a practical benefit from the research. Through modern technology the equipment may become as affordable as a home computer, and thus become a more popular treatment for neuromuscular disabilities.

Biofeedback is based on the fact that electrical impulses generated by an active muscle can be received and retransmitted to the patient in the form of audible or visible signals. Often a few active motor units remain in paralyzed muscles, including that part of the nerve from the spinal cord to the muscle fiber it affects. The weak electrical impulses generated by the muscle's activity can guide the patient's exercise program by indicating muscle contraction so slight that no visual motion occurs. When a patient exercises with the EMM as a guide, the activity sometimes spreads to other muscle fibers, the muscle fibers sometimes grow stronger, and the whole muscle sometimes becomes stronger.

Muscle contraction occurs when the brain sends electrical signals to the muscles through the nerves. The impulses start in the brain, travel through the spinal cord, pass across the nerves, and finally reach the muscle. Muscle fibers group together to make up muscle bundles, with many bundles forming each muscle.

When there is an injury, impulses from the brain can be "short-circuited." If the injury is extensive and impulses cannot get through to the muscle at all, paralysis occurs. Usually the muscles begin to atrophy after three weeks of paralysis and permanent damage may occur. Although passive range-of-motion exercises can prevent muscle atrophy, they are important in maintaining the flexibility of joints in these cases.

Any electrical activity of the muscle can be picked up by the EMM. The impulses recorded are generated by muscle fiber contraction, not by the nerves. The slightest activity can be identified and the degree of dysfunction ascertained. Even when a muscle seems to be totally paralyzed, there often remain a few active motor units. Along with these there are latent motor units which can sometimes be reactivated by exercise. Often good nerves can take over more muscle fibers to develop larger motor units. Muscles that were once paralyzed may function again, even though they may never be as strong as they once were and may tire easily.

In 1968, Marinacci noted the following:

"The most important factors in neuromuscular reeducation or reactivation of the motor units are an increase in the voltage, the duration, the frequency, and the promptness of the motor unit's response to voluntary efforts. These results are best obtained from the development of physiological compensatory factors as seen in the formation of the giant motor units. Motor units have been observed to increase in voltage from about 0.5 microvolts to as much as 25 microvolts. This may increase in duration from 5 to 30 milliseconds within a period of twelve to eighteen months."[1]

Today the results are more astounding. You may see a head injured patient, previously confined to a wheelchair, walking without the aid of braces or crutches. The techniques used in treatment have become more sophisticated yet simplified. A television monitor receives signals by way of electrodes attached to certain parts of the body, and measures the motor signals from the brain to specific muscles. When the signal gets through to the correct muscle, dots on the TV screen move toward the top of the screen. This visual information substitutes for the missing natural feedback from the muscles.

In other words, those head injured patients who suffer from serious gait (walking) difficulties or hand control problems can learn to correctly contract the proper muscles for movement. Once the patient has learned the correct pattern of motor commands, he may be able to move the affected limbs without being attached to the feedback machine.

Using the biofeedback machine successfully involves a process called operant conditioning (trial-and-error learning). The technique is very flexible; correct responses are rewarded and thereby strengthened, or learned. In this case, the reward is seeing the dot move up on the TV screen and thus realizing that the muscle is being controlled by the patient. The patient's self-esteem grows as success becomes obvious.

One young boy who had been in an auto accident at age three suffered head injury and could not move his right hand and arm. After nine years of rigorous physical therapy, the wrist and fingers remained spastic and uncontrollable. After 10 biofeedback sessions within two weeks, the boy had learned to grasp a glass and lift it to his mouth, to use a fork, and to use his right arm and hand for eating, dressing, and other everyday activities!

Victims previously resigned to spending their lives in wheelchairs are now walking. The results are startling and are now achieving public attention. Recently a television documentary on drunk driving was seen nationally. One victim of an auto accident was head injured, but was able to walk again through the use of biofeedback. Such public attention can encourage the use of this technique and create a demand for treatment throughout the country, not just on a local basis.

9. Proposing new ideas that appear to have potential. I am suggesting for consideration a therapeutic approach that has just recently been used to treat victims of head trauma, particularly in the California area where it originated. There appears to be just cause to believe that it may be helpful. This technique is called "sensory integration."

First I should like to present some information obtained through the Bay Area Association for Sensory Integration in Albany, California. In one of their booklets, "Sensory Integration: Information for Parents," based on work by Dr. A. Jean Ayres, they give information for parents of children with learning disabilities, but you will probably note the similarities to head injury.

Before discussing sensory integration we must know precisely what it is. To put it simply, sensory integration is the ability to take in, sort out, and connect information from the world around us. The central nervous system (including nerves, the spinal cord, and the brain) controls this process. Our senses take in this information, transmitting it to the brain by way of the nerves and spinal cord. In normal circumstances our understanding of what is sensed is automatic.

When our sensory integrative powers are working properly, we are protected from danger and are able to interact and learn from our environment. When the system is not working properly, the patient usually exhibits severe behavior problems because of frustration. In more technical terms the process is as follows:

"The brain receives vast amounts of information from each of our senses. This sensory information stimulates the nervous system to produce body movements, thoughts, and feelings, which are fundamentals of our personality and self-image. As a child learns to move his body, balance himself, and relate to the objects and people around him, his brain organizes the incoming sensory information. This organization — which is called 'sensory integration' — enables us to direct our attention, to produce useful and well-coordinated behavior, and to feel okay about ourselves.

"In the first seven or eight years of life, a child develops the brain organzation which will be the foundation for his later learning and behavior. In these early years, the spontaneous movements of play involving the entire body are most effective in developing the nervous system.

"In some children, the brain is not able to organize certain sensations. Therefore, these sensations interfere with the child's learning and behavior. The child sees and hears and feels, but some of this information does not 'make sense' to him. He does not learn properly from this information and will not be able to deal effectively with his environment. These children usually show some combination of the following problems (particularly keep in mind here the problems with victims of head trauma and see how they compare):

1. Lack of strength and firmness in the muscles. This may result in poor posture and fatigue.

2. A poor sense of balance, so that the child may be insecure in standing and in moving.

3. Lack of coordination between the two sides of the body. The child may be clumsy and confused when he has to use both hands or both feet together.

4. Lack of coordination between the eyes and the body, so that the child does not effectively use visual information to assist him in his actions.

5. Poor attention span. The child often has difficulty focusing on a task.

6. Confusion on performing an unfamiliar sequence of skilled movements. The child can handle a new task only if he thinks about each movement.

7. Overactive behavior and restlessness. The child has difficulty responding in a relaxed yet alert manner. He reacts as though compelled to do so. This problem is sometimes called hyperactivity.

8. A poorly developed sense of touch, and sometimes discomfort when touched. The child may have difficulty learning the shape and texture of things.

9. Difficulty using and understanding language . . . problems in speaking, reading, and writing.

"In general, the child has difficulty both in play and in work. He may not succeed along with his peers, or he has to use so much effort that he does not enjoy himself. He has trouble with personal relationships because he cannot relax and pay attention to another person . . . directing and controlling the incoming sensory stimuli through sensory integrative therapy, children are able to learn more effectively at home, school, and play.

"This process of reorganizing the brain does not involve drugs or complex equipment, nor does it require psychotherapy or medical treatment. Sensory integration therapy relies upon the natural sensory experience which occurs in body activities. Instead of making new demands on the family or teaching, or trying to force the child to behave, sensory integration therapy enhances the child's ability to learn and to adapt.

"Sensory integration therapy is given by an occupational therapist or physical therapist who has had additional training in nervous system function and sensory integration. The child is given a series of standardized tests which indicate his level of sensory integrative ability. Since the brain develops in an orderly sequence, the therapist must follow that sequence starting with the child's most basic difficulty. Each child is unique, and the therapy is structured for that child's individual needs . . . (Specific activities) produce improvement at each level of nervous system development. These activities usually involve the entire body and many senses at once. They require skillful yet spontaneous body responses, since sensory integration occurs without deliberate concentration. On the surface, it may appear that the child in sensory integration therapy is merely playing or doing exercises. However, the therapist has organized the environment and the child's activities so that his sensory network is stimulated in the most effective way. Because of therapy the child's nervous system now begins allowing him to learn."[1]

Specific techniques relating to balance, movement, and touch improve one's senses, originating in the brain stem, from early childhood to more complete development. Sensory integration is most likely to occur when the child enjoys the activity and feels satisfied in reaching a new level of success. Therefore, the child should feel challenged when he first approaches the activity. As he adapts to this challenge, his brain organizes itself for greater efficiency. There is less effort and stress, and the child is free to enjoy himself.

"A child's sense of fulfillment radiates as he experiences himself interacting affectively with the world of objects, or as he pits himself against gravity and finds that it is not quite the ruthless master it was a short time before, or as he finds his body bringing him satisfying sensation. He is no longer the impotent organism shoved about by environmental forces; he can act effectively on the world. He is more of a whole being."[1]

Let us look as this technique in respect to head trauma. The key word is "child." Sensory integration has proved quite successful with various learning disabilities symptomatically similar to those occurring with head injury. True, head injury is characterized by other identifiable symptoms, but it appears that the brain dysfunction may be originating from the same site. As we have seen in Chapters 7 and 8, physical and occupational therapists use specific standardized techniques and equipment to improve balance, walking, coordination, as well as cognition. Likewise, sensory integration is organized according to the child's level of competence. Let us take this one step further. Why stop at the boundaries of traditional physical and occupational therapy?

Even during coma, the techniques of sensory integration could be effective. Touching, massaging, rolling, sitting up, movement, and verbal stimuli are already recognized as helpful even when the patient does not appear to be conscious of his surroundings. Later, as the patient emerges from the coma, the therapist can continue with more sophisticated techniques, depending on the patient's physical condition. The playlike atmosphere would seem to be conducive to learning in the childlike mind of the victim of head trauma. This therapy can be used in conjunction with other therapies in a team program to achieve maximum success.

Imagine an inflated vinyl ball, large enough to support an adult. By lying on the ball, the patient, under close supervision of course, must learn to stay on it without falling. He learns about his body — how to move it to achieve balance, how one movement can result in falling off, how another movement causes rocking, and so forth. Even on a simpler level, rolling on the floor can be used to familiarize the patient with body movement. Almost every victim of head trauma has to use the tilt board and parallel bars at some time in therapy; the movements used in sensory integration carry this idea one step further.

Instead of putting a round peg into a round hole to help in recognizing spatial differences, the patient may crawl through an obstacle course of various rubber or vinyl shapes. Shapes are perceived on a larger-than-life basis just as gross motor skills are improved before fine motor skills. Instead of showing a patient cards with various shapes on them (stars, hearts, circles, crosses, or letters, for example), the shapes are three dimensional. The patient must feel the shape, out of view, and try to identify that shape from a selection that he can see. The pictures become real, tangible things that he can relate to more readily. As the processes of the brain improve, the learning progresses to more complex tasks. All the senses are employed to facilitate understanding and make the patient feel better about himself.

While I was observing physical and occupational therapy for quite a few head trauma patients, what I was learning about sensory integration seemed to fit right in. I was motivated to investigate the specific processes involved with sensory integrative development and found startling similarities with what I already knew about head injury.

The entire process is broken down into four blocks, the first being the receiving of input through the senses. The tactile sense (referring to touch) is made up of a protective system that alerts the body to heat, cold, and so forth and a discriminative system that identifies hardness, softness, roughness, and smoothness. When this area in a head injured person is damaged, he is in great danger of harming himself.

Another sense is the vestibular (or balance) mechanism of the body. In the head injured victim, the tilt table and parallel bars are used to directly deal with this problem. Especially early in rehabilitation, many patients have difficulty in controlling where they are in relationship to the enrivonment.

Closely related to balance are the proprioceptors, which give us information from our muscles, tendons, ligaments, and joints about the position of our body parts. Often there may be no physical damage, yet the patient may not be able to move an arm or a leg.

The senses of smell (olfactory), taste, sight, and hearing also fit into this block. In my case the nerves that receive taste and smell stimuli were destroyed, and there was no way to regain these senses. However, I have noted in many patients that these senses were severely affected during the early stages of recovery. Through the healing process, however, these senses returned, obviously because there had merely been a shock to the nerve, not destruction of it.

The second block in the sensory integrative process involves the body and movement. The "body scheme" lets us recognize the position of all our body parts as well as their potential for movement. It is the job of the brain to integrate the stimuli brought to it by the sensory system described in block 1 and make the individual aware of this scheme.

"Reflex maturation" refers to the development of automatic movements or reflexes such as the knee jerk. These reflexes must give way to complex voluntary movement so that the body can effectively overcome gravity. As these reflexes mature, they diminish in intensity so that our motor skills can take over.

The capacity to screen sensory input is important because we are constantly being bombarded by stimuli. Unless irrelevant stimuli are screened out, the patient cannot focus on a task or respond appropriately.

Also in block 2 is the process of achieving postural security, awareness of two sides of our body, and motor planning. Postural security, sometimes referred to as being "earth bound," refers to feeling secure about moving and changing positions. The awareness of two sides of the body relates to the patient's ability to make both sides work together as well as to recognize the differences. I did not know left from right until the idea was "drilled" into me by constant repetition. Many patients have difficulty in coordinating movements between the two sides of the body and therefore need exercises to improve their recognition of this problem.

Finally, motor planning is the ability to think through a new motor task. By knowing our "body scheme," we integrate the sensory information received by the brain and order our body parts to respond. Learning to jump rope, as I did, involves this process of motor planning.

Blocks 1 and 2 lay the foundation of our perceptual motor skills described as block 3. These include eye-hand coordination, oculomotor control (reading), postural adjustments (required to perform fine and gross motor tasks), auditory language skills (understanding and using speech), visual spatial perception (awareness of form and space), and attention center functions (screening stimuli).

Finally, in block 4, the brain carries out the process of learning and emotional response. When there is a dysfunction, a patient cannot learn from previous experiences. This could be either the result of an inadequate sensory integrative system or the effect of short term memory loss. Here is the basis for later academic learning. The techniques for the treatment of this problem are the same no matter what the cause.

One of our goals in treating the head injured patient is to provide the tools for learning as well as improve the conceptual ability to learn, in the hope that both will finally work automatically. Exercises are used to improve the use of the tools we need for learning, especially in the areas of reading; hand-eye coordination; the learning of letters, numbers, and words; the remembering of symbols and letters placed in order for spelling; and the learning of mathematical concepts.

I must remind the reader that sensory integration is only one technique, admittedly untested, that seems to have the potential for being beneficial in the treatment of head trauma. Others are being employed at various rehabilitation centers and are gaining recognition as effective procedures.

Response:

Sensory integration does indeed appear to have promise as an effective treatment approach with the head injured patient. Many therapists have already been using a modified sensory integrative approach with good success. For additional information on this unique approach, the reader is referred to the references.[2,3,4]

—*Barbara Zoltan*

There are other techniques now being employed which are not so beneficial. I feel that it is important here to warn the families of head injured patients about the get-rich schemes that are presently appearing in the wake of public awareness of head trauma. Some therapists, looking for an easy way to cash in on this awareness, are opening rehabilitation centers utilizing some techniques standard to occupational or recreational therapy and advertising them as "wonder treatments" for victims of head trauma. They are doing nothing new, nothing not already being done presently in rehabilitation centers to integrate other forms of therapy into the patient's treatment. Members of the victim's family must be wary in selecting an appropriate rehabilitation center by finding out exactly what methods of treatment are used there.

Let your voice be heard. Write your Congressman, organize meetings, speak to the press, and do anything else that will make this silent epidemic "come out of the closet." Federal support is crucial if nationwide recognition is to be achieved and action taken.

Many actions are currently being taken to change things. On a local level, legislation has been introduced in New Jersey to help victims of head trauma. In 1984 an act was introduced to provide an appropriation of $75,000 to establish a demonstration day rehabilitation program within the state Department of Human Services, and a law signed in April 1985 created the Division of Developmental Disabilities to provide services to the non-mentally retarded and developmentally disabled, including certain head injured persons.

The recognition of head injury as a real problem has opened the door to further legislation, and other states (as well as the federal government) are now beginning to follow suit.

The provisions of the New Jersey bill include the following:
1. a comprehensive, statewide needs assessment,
2. outreach services,
3. professional training for personnel of the Division of Developmental Disabilities,
4. a media campaign emphasizing prevention, and
5. recommendations to provide comprehensive service.

In addition, the Commissioner of the Department of Human Services is required to report to the governor and the legislature on the findings of the needs assessment no later than August 1987. To implement this, the Division's Office of Grants Management will be responsible for contracting with the New Jersey Head Injury Association. Other offices will work to ensure that the outreach and professional training activities are closely coordinated with regional offices' efforts to provide services for the head injured.

Another bill introduced recently would establish and maintain a central registry for persons who have sustained head injuries. The purpose is to ascertain the medical and rehabilitative needs of the population so that better health care can be provided. Once this information is compiled, the government can work on providing rehabilitation services for these victims.

On a national level, fact-finding committees are busy gathering information so that federal legislation can be provided. Public interest can help greatly in making head injury a subject that is familiar and obviously in need of action.

Other areas of legislation are also affected by the recognition of head trauma as an epidemic. No-fault insurance laws are now being reevaluated in many states. Many motorists wish to abolish these laws, not realizing that the premiums will not necessarily be lowered as benefits are reduced. Those involved with head trauma feel that abolishing no-fault insurance would have adverse effects in cases of catastrophic injury. Because there is often a long wait for settlement, public funding must cover interim costs in states where no-fault insurance is not available. There is also usually a cap on medical liability, which affects those victims requiring long-term treatment. Furthermore, there is no provision for treatment which is not required until many years after the injury.

For example, the current no-fault system in New Jersey is very unbalanced, allowing unlimited medical coverage and a $200 threshold for liability suits. The local Head Injury Foundation proposes that the present system be modified to include unlimited medical coverage, and balanced by limiting the liability threshold to a verbal threshhold (liability suits would be limited to cases of serious impairment of body function, permanent serious disfigurement, or death).

This is just one example of a phenomenon sweeping aross the country. Many state legislatures are introducing laws to enforce the use of seat belts or the installation of air bags in cars. Those states which already have seat belt laws are publicizing statistics which encourage other states to follow suit. Although such laws have only been in effect for a short time, fatalities and critical injuries has dramatically decreased already.

Independent studies are also determining which cars are safest in respect to head injuries. By driving well-constructed cars, using seat belts, and being more aware of defensive driving, motorists can significantly reduce the frequency and serious of accidents.

This chapter began with the question, "What's next?" I see a bright future for head trauma treatment. Present and future victims will benefit from the actions being taken nationwide to advance this cause. So what will happen to the Davids and Marys and all the others described in this book?

David will be able to get a job that he enjoys and finds emotionally rewarding. Perhaps he will be dealing with head injured patients in a rehabilitation setting. If not, he will find work with an employer who understands head injury enough to recognize David's positive contribution to the work force.

Brian will continue to develop and improve. With maturity, many of his problems may disappear. He is capable of leading a "normal" life because of his acceptance of his disability. Likewise, Jerry, Darren, and Nancy will be able to return to happy and productive lives almost as though nothing had happened. I hope that they will accept and understand their experiences and use that knowledge to help others who would benefit from their inspirational stories.

There is hope for Mary also, who could become more self-sufficient in a group home setting where she can develop to her full potential. She may not be able to function independently, but that does not mean that her life cannot be rewarding.

The case of Nick is sad because the hope for improvement is so dim. Perhaps he can serve as a living warning against drunk driving and the value of life that can so easily be destroyed in an instant. Nick's suffering and that of his family were avoidable. Public awareness is the first step in decreasing the unfortunate statistics involving head injury.

I can visualize head trauma centers across the country dedicated solely to the care and treatment of victims of head trauma. Programs will be developed integrating a multitude of techniques. Every head injured person will benefit from the efforts of persistent families and professionals who are dedicated to improving the quality of life for all. Victims who are alone will find those who care. Families who are lost will find the support and understanding of others who have been there. We are surely on the threshold of a new era of understanding and treatment of head injuries. Just as man awakened from the ignorance of the Stone Age with the discovery of fire, 20th Century man is awakening from the ignorance of the Nuclear Age with a glimmer of understanding of the brain and human capabilities. If we can send men to the moon and beyond, we can surely combat ignorance.

Response:
Many facilities dedicated solely to the care of head injury patients have already opened. Presently there are approximately 400 facilites nationwide. These centers range in scope of care from care for the comatose to subacute rehabilitation, and from transitional living arrangements to day treatment programs.

—*Barbara Zoltan*

The candle flickers,
At first uncertain, barely seen.
One voice sings alone.
The gentle wind feeds the flame
As other voices join the song.
We shall not curse the darkness,
But let the brightness of our love
Encircle all with choruses of joy.

—Beverly Slater

References

1. Owen S, Toomin H, Taylor, LP: Biofeedback in Neuromuscular Re-Education. Biofeedback Research Institute, Inc., 1975.

2. Siev E, Freishtat B, Zoltan B: Perceptual and Cognitive Dysfunction of the Adult Stroke Patient. Thorofare, NJ, Slack, Inc., 1986.

3. Ayres AJ: Sensory Integration and Learning Disorders. Los Angeles, CA, Western Psychological Services, 1980.

4. Ayres AJ: Sensory Integration and the Child. Los Angeles, CA, Western Psychological Services, 1979.

APPENDIX A

Appendix A: PHARMACOLOGIC INTERACTIONS PERTINENT TO HEAD INJURY PATIENTS

Name	Purpose	Contraindications	Side Effects	Comments
Elavil®	Antidepressant Level II/III to heighten arousal; with higher levels to decrease agitation	Arrhythmias Urinary retention	Change in BP, change in blood sugar, sweating, dry mouth, weakness, fatigue, tingling, tremors, ataxia, arrhythmias, initial sedation, breast enlargement or testicular swelling	Is a central nervous system depressant which acts to decrease psychological depression
Tofranil®	Antidepressant	Myocaridal infarction	Change in blood pressure, confusional states, numbness, tingling, ataxia, tremors, dry mouth, blurred vision, change in blood sugar	Stimulation of central nervous system
Ritalin®	CNS stimulation to heighten alertness	Hypertension, history of drug dependency	Ataxia, insomnia, cardiac arrhythmia, nausea, anorexia, blurred vision, skin rash	Monitor blood pressure, "tolerance" to drug effect
Phenobarbital	Anticonvulsant (seizure prevention)	Severe trauma, severe hypotension, uncontrolled diabetes, drug dependence	Lethargy/sedation, skin rash, ataxia, nystagmus, osteomalacia, habit-forming	Drug discontinuance should be done gradually
Thorazine®	Tranquilization Management of psychotic disorders	Comatose states Presence of large amounts of CNS depressants	Drowsiness, jaundice, hypotension (usually transient), neuromuscular extrapyramidal reactions, dystonias, pseudoparkinsonism, potential for hepatotoxicity	Precise mechanisms unknown

Appendix A (continued)

Name	Purpose	Contraindications	Side Effects	Comments
Haldol®	Tranquilization Management of psychotic disorders	Severe toxic CNS depression or comatose states Parkinson's disease	Neuromuscular extrapyramidal reactions, Parkinson-like symptoms, restlessness, dystonia, Akathisia, drowsiness	Dopamine blocker
Mellaril®	Tranquilization Management of manifestations of psychotic disorders	Severe CNS depression or comatose strokes	Drowsiness, infrequently Extrapyramidal symptoms	
Navane®	Tranquilization Management of manifestations of psychotic disorders	Patients with circulatory collapse, comatose states, CNS depression, blood dyscrosias	Drowsiness, restlessness, agitation	May precipitate convulsions
Artane®	Adjunct in treatment of all forms of Parkinsonism Control of extrapyramidal disorders caused by CNS drugs	Cautious use for patients with cardiac, liver or kidney disorders or with hypertension	Dryness of mouth, blurring of vision, dizziness, mild nausea or nervousness	Size and frequency of dosage to control extrapyramidal reactions to tranquilizers must be determined empirically
Dilantin®	Anticonvulsant	Previous hypersensitivity	Skin rash, hyperglycemia, osteomalacia, nystagmus, ataxia, gum hyperplasia	Drug discontinuance should be done gradually

Appendix A (continued)

Name	Purpose	Contraindications	Side Effects	Comments
Tegretol®	Anticonvulsant temporal lobe	Liver abnormality	CBC abnormalities, rash, cardiac effects, (arrhythmia, edema, CHF) sedation	Long term therapy is associated with hepatic complications
Dantrium®	To control spasticity	Liver abnormalities	Drowsiness, dizziness, weakness, fatigue, diarrhea Potential for Hepatotoxicity (with greater than 800 mg daily)	Discontinue if no change in 45 days Directly interferes with the contractile mechanism of the muscle
Lioresal® (Ballofen)	To control spasticity General CNS depressant	Diabetes, Epilepsy (should be monitored)	Transient drowsiness, dizziness, fatigue, frequent urge to urinate, constipation, nausea, impaired renal function	Should not exceed 80 mg/d Abrupt withdrawal can lead to hallucinations (interferes with the release of excitatory transmitters)
Valium®	To control spasticity Skeletal muscle relaxant	Children under 6 months of age	Drowsiness, fatigue, ataxia, headaches, confusion, depression, blurred vision, or double vision, skin rashes, urinary incontinence, constipation	May enhance effectiveness of Dilantin Physical/psychological dependence Lowers blood pressure

Developed by: Marion Miller, RPT
For: New England Rehabilitation Hospital
    Brain Injury Unit
    Orientation Packet for Staff Physical Therapists
Orientation Packet, compiled by: Marion Miller, RPT and Mary Evens, RPT

APPENDIX B
QUESTIONS FOR FAMILIES TO ASK WHEN LOOKING FOR A REHABILITATION FACILITY

First, be sure to call ahead and ask if you can visit the facility and ask if anyone would be available to give you a tour or answer the following questions:

1. Does the facility have a separate head trauma unit? How does the unit address the specific cognitive, behavioral, and physical needs of the head trauma population, and of your family member in particular?

2. What is the ratio of nurses to patients?

3. Is there a trained team of therapists, nurses, and physicians who have expertise in head trauma rehabilitation? Do these remain consistent, i.e., does the patient have the same nurse or therapist every day? Are social workers, neuropsychologists, vocational and recreational specialists part of the team?

4. How much treatment is provided daily? How often is it provided by each therapy discipline—once, twice daily? Is treatment delivered on a one-to-one basis or in groups?

5. Visit the treatment environment—is it a separate, quiet room?

6. Are physicians and psychiatrists accessible to speak with you personally or on the phone? Are the staff on full time?

7. What are the common medications given head trauma patients? Are patients medicated if agitated or depressed?

8. Can arrangements be made for consultations—ophthalmology, gynecology, dermatology, dental, podiatric, orthotic, orthopedics, etc.

9. Is the social worker familiar with your insurance and with community services for head trauma victims?

10. Does the facility's program include out-trips, day passes, or overnights to assist with the patient's transition to the outside world—or does the facility offer any therapeutic extras such as a pool or a driving evaluation?

11. What are the visiting hours for family and friends?

12. What is seen as the family's role in the patient's rehabilitation?

13. Does the facility offer family conferences, family education classes, or individual or family counseling?

14. Where do visitors park? What is the cost, if any?

15. Can affordable arrangements be made close to the facility for family members who live out of town to stay at while the patient is in the hospital?

16. Does the facility offer an out-patient program geared specifically to head trauma patients? If so, is transportation available.

—Maria Kendricken, BS, RPT

APPENDIX C
BEHAVIORAL MANAGEMENT STRATEGIES

Problems in the area of behavior are often present in patients who have sustained an injury to the brain. Behavior problems may be a direct result of the injury, occur as a secondary effect, or as an exaggeration of premorbid personality traits. Behavior problems tend to interfere with all aspects of therapy and tend to endure over time.

Behavior Problems

Aggression:
a. Verbal: shout obscenities and insults
b. Physical: striking out at a person or at the environment

Sexual Provocation:
a. Verbal: harassment and/or inappropriate seductive comments or jokes.
b. Physical: exposing genitals or masturbation. Inappropriate touching of others.

Social disinhibition:
Poor control of impulses in social situations. Lack of social judgment in conversation, e.g., rude or insulting comments or gestures. Overfamiliarity (verbal or physical). General lack of awareness of how behavior affects others.

Denial:
Blaming others for deficits or lack of progress. Also, aggressive behaviors or refusal to participate in Rx.

Depression:
Despondency, apathy, passive/aggressive behaviors, neglecting one's self-care (eating, hygiene), tearful.

Agitation/Irritability:
Impatience, restlessness, low frustration tolerance, disagreeable, combative with little provocation.

Passivity/Dependency:
Low self-esteem, following therapist around, requires excessive positive reinforcement, childlike dependency; asks for permission to do things. May show "poor me" attitude.

Treatment Strategies

1. Consistency is the key in reducing disruptive behavior. It establishes predictability for the patient. For example, treat in the same environment. Give consistent responses to behavior. Have a consistent primary and covering therapist. Use a consistent schedule, explaining what is going to happen and why if appropriate.

2. Gear treatment towards positive experiences. At times it may be necessary to begin and end sessions which provide less challenge to the patient. This would allow for a successful experience especially important for patients who show depression, low frustration tolerance, or passivity.

3. Set firm limits and give patient clear feedback about the effect of his behavior on others. Allow for role playing or repeating the situation, so that patients may receive a positive response from their environment.

4. Attempt to give the patient some control over treatment planning by offering choices of therapeutic activities and by allowing for breaks or time out as needed. Build responsibility into the treatment program to increase investment and self-esteem. Avoid power struggles.

5. Whenever possible incorporate patient's interests in an attempt to promote self-motivation and investment in treatment.

6. Do not force the patient to remain in an uncomfortable environment. Switching treatment environments may be appropriate.

7. Avoid surprises, quick movements, unanticipated or uncomfortable touching. Warn the patient when a treatment modality may be painful or noxious.

8. A familiar contact may be helpful in extreme phases of agitation or irritability, or simply to increase patient cooperation in treatment.

9. Attempt to reduce stimulation for the patient by responding in a calm voice, which should be consistent with body language.

10. Redirect patient's attention away from source or cause of frustration.

11. Be careful of your body language. Be aware of patient's ego boundaries or concept of personal body space.

12. Either write or verbally contract with patient prior to treatment which behaviors are permissible and which are not. Include length of time specific behaviors will be required.

Developed by: Charlene Arthur Greirard, OTR-L and Jane Kenig, OTR-L
For: New England Rehabilitation Hospital Brain Injury Unit
Orientation Packet for Staff Physical Therapists
Compiled by Marion Miller, RTP and Mary Evens, RPT

APPENDIX D
ACTIVE SUPPORT GROUPS IN PENNSYLVANIA

Eastern Pennsylvania

Allentown. Meets the second Sunday of every month at 2 p.m. at Good Shepherd Rehabilitation Hospital. Contact Carol Gober, 215-264-0154.

Bucks County. Meets the first Thursday of every month at St. Mary Hospital, Langhorne, at 7:30 p.m. Contact Betty Tomlinson, 215-945-1115.

Camp Hill. Meets the second Tuesday of every month at 10 a.m. at 2117 Mayfred Lane. Contact Shirley Coombe, 717-737-2497.

Danville. Meets the third Tuesday of every month at 7:30 p.m. in the Neurophysiology Laboratory Waiting Room at Geisinger Medical Center. Contact Sharon Smeltz, 814-349-5307 or 814-238-3139.

Doylestown. Meets on alternate Wednesdays from 5:30 to 7 p.m. in Conference Room F at the Doylestown Hospital Rehabilitation Center. Contact Lana Liberto, 215-345-2609.

Elizabethtown. Meets the third Wednesday of every month at 8 p.m. in the Physical Therapy Gymnasium of Elizabethtown Hospital. Contact Gayle Barney, 717-367-1161.

Elwyn. Meets the last Thursday of every month at 7:30 p.m. at the Elwyn Institute. Contact Nadine Colgan or Lynn Vosbikian, 215-358-6711.

Malvern. Meets the second Tuesday of every month at 7 p.m. at Bryn Mawr Rehabilitation Hospital. Contact Terri Monachese, 215-251-5400.

Mechanicsburg. Meets the third Saturday of every month at 11 a.m. at the Rehabilitation Hospital, 4950 Wilson Lane. Contact Linda Hammer, 717-697-8211, extension 304.

Milford (Scranton area). Meets the second Saturday of every month at noon at Hillcrest, 404 E. Harford Street. Contact Mary Girardi or Tony McCormack, 717-296-9261.

Philadelphia. Hospital of the University of Pennsylvania. Meets the first Thursday of every month at 7 p.m. in the Ravdin Building, 5th floor, room 1514, 3400 Spruce Street. For information call 215-662-3486.

Philadelphia. Magee Rehabilitation Hospital, Six Franklin Plaza. Meets the second Thursday of every month at 6:30 p.m. Contact Elaine McGarry, 609-428-1210, or Sue Apter, 215-665-5100.

Reading. Meets the third Thursday of every month at 7 p.m. at Reading Rehabilitation Hospital. Contact Mary Anne Ohlinger, 215-929-8315.

Tioga. Meets the third Thursday of every month at 7:30 p.m. in the Broad Acres Activity Room, Wellsboro, Pa. Contact Janice Davis, 717-835-5144, or Julie Albough, 717-724-1857.

Wilkes-Barre. Meets the third Thursday of every month at 7 p.m. at the Wilkes-Barre General Hospital. Contact Roseanne Carroll, 717-824-2432.

Williamsport. Meets the first Monday of every month at 7:30 p.m. in the Second Rehabilitation Dining Room at Williamsport Hospital. Contact Glenn W. Thompson, 717-321-2661.

York. Meets the first and third Tuesdays of every month at 7 p.m. at the Rehabilitation Hospital of York. Contact Michelle Zimmerman, 717-767-6941, extension 723.

Western Pennsylvania

Altoona. Meets the fourth Wednesday of every month at 7 p.m. at the Howard Avenue Medical Center, Building C. Contact Bruce Strittmatter, 814-674-8098.

Beaver. Meets at various times at the Easter Seal Society Building, Dutch Ridge Road. Contact Marland Weiss, 412-378-1991 (evenings only).

Erie. Meets at various times and locations. Contact Annie Bogda, 814-474-3379.

Pittsburgh. Meets the first Tuesday of every month at VRC, 1323 Forbes Avenue. Contact Joyce Schlag, 412-741-9500.

Uniontown. Meets at various times and locations. Contact Marcia Cohen, 412-438-0343.

Westmoreland. Meets the second Wednesday of every month. Contact Verna Smith, 412-872-6610 or 412-539-1488.

Currently additional support groups are being organized in the Johnstown, Washington, and Erie areas.

APPENDIX E
FAMILY HEAD
TRAUMA
QUESTIONNAIRE

Because you are a relative of a head trauma victim, your comments will be most valuable in formulating a program to benefit both victims and families of victims. Please answer the following questions. Sometimes a yes-or-no answer will be suitable and sometimes a brief explanation will be necessary. Thank you for your kind cooperation.

1. What is your relationship to the patient?

2. What caused the head trauma?

3. In what year did the accident occur?

4. When you received news of the accident, did you know whom to call for information?

5. Did you have any say in the emergency treatment of the patient?

6. Was long term parking made available for you and your relatives at the hospital?

7. Was someone immediately available for you and your relatives to speak with when you arrived at the hospital?

8. Were you allowed liberal or unlimited visiting privileges?

9. Was physical therapy given during coma? If "yes," what was done?

10. Were you told precisely what to expect in regard to medical procedures?

11. Was the topic of "brain damage" discussed or even thought of in the beginning?

12. Were the doctors and nurses positive, negative, or noncommittal about recovery?

13. Was someone available to discuss insurance and legal matters with you and your family?

14. Were you told about the specific procedures to be used by each therapist and doctor?

15. Was the patient examined by a psychologist or a psychiatrist?

16. Was counseling available for the patient?

17. Was counseling available for the family?

18. Were you encouraged to help in the therapy (e.g., occupational therapy, physical therapy)?

19. Was there a team effort among the therapists, or did each one work independently? Was the family involved?

20. Was the nursing care adequate?

21. Who was responsible for the greatest progress — the nurses, the therapists, or the family?

22. Was the daily routine performed by primary nurses, or by licensed practical nurses?

23. Was the primary nurse aware of the patient's progress, or was her case load too great for her to give close attention?

24. If the patient was the breadwinner of the family, did you receive any help in solving future financial problems?

25. If the patient was a child, was schooling available during rehabilitation?

26. Was any effort made to determine the mental age of the patient?

27. If "yes," was the patient treated like a child of that age?

28. Did the patient suffer long term or short term memory loss?

29. Was there a personality change in the patient? If "yes," please describe briefly:

30. Who seemed to have the most difficulty in adjusting to the injury — the patient, the parents, children, or siblings?

31. What gave the patient the greatest sense of accomplishment?

32. Was there a great deal of physical damage other than the head trauma?

33. Did you get any help from a social worker or another source in choosing the best rehabilitation facility for the patient?

34. Aside from physical limitations, what was the greatest problem to overcome?

35. Did you participate in any of the therapy sessions with the patient?

36. Did you work with the patient after therapy time (evenings and weekends)?

37. Did you have to work with the patient on your own, or were you encouraged by the therapists to do so?

38. Was the patient allowed home on weekends from rehabilitation? If "yes," did the patient and the family react in a positive way? Did the patient want to go back to the hospital after these visits?

39. How did the patient react to physical therapy (positively, negatively, or neutrally)?

40. How did the patient react to occupational therapy (positively, negatively, or neutrally)?

41. How did the patient react to other types of therapy (e.g., speech, recreational)?

42. Did lack of progress in one area affect progress in other areas?

43. What was the single greatest adjustment the family had to make in response to the patient's head trauma?

The following six questions are directed at those whose relative has been released from the inpatient rehabilitation unit and is living at home or on his own:

44. Upon discharge from the rehabilitation center what did the patient do? Return to work? Return to school? Retrain for another job? Other?

45. Was there a need for further therapy or counseling after discharge?

46. If the head trauma occurred prior to 1984, has the situation changed? If "yes," how?

47. How does the patient feel about his future (positive, negative, or noncommittal)?

48. How do you feel about the future (positive, negative, or noncommittal)?

49. Would you have benefited from a book about understanding and treating head trauma had it been available when the accident occurred?

50. Please briefly suggest improvements that should be made or techniques you may have improvised that proved successful and that could help others. If you think of other questions that would be useful in this survey, please include them here.

APPENDIX F
VICTIM HEAD TRAUMA QUESTIONNAIRE

As a victim of head trauma, your input will be most valuable in the formulation of a program to benefit both other victims and their families. Please answer the following questions as completely as possible. Thank you for your kind cooperation.

1. Was your head injury a result of a motor vehicle accident?
2. In what year did it happen?
3. What is your age now?
4. Who was the first person to be notified about the accident?
5. Were you taken to a trauma center? Other location?
6. Who was the first person you remember seeing?
7. Do you remember anything about the hospital after the crisis? If "yes," what?
8. Did you know why you were in the hospital at first?
9. Do you remember events before your head trauma?
10. Do you have trouble with short term memory?
11. Do you remember physical therapy?
12. Do you remember occupational therapy?
13. What problem was the most difficult for you during rehabiliation?
14. Do friends treat you differently now?
15. Who helped you the most?
16. Was there any therapy that was a waste of time? If "yes," what was it?
17. What therapy did you dislike most?
18. Which therapy did you enjoy the most?
19. What therapy was the most useful?
20. Would a book about understanding and treating head trauma be helpful for your family, yourself, and therapists?

You may use the remaining space to write any comments or suggestions.

GLOSSARY OF TERMS

Abstraction. A general idea or word representing a concrete concept.

Activities of daily living (ADL). Include dressing, feeding, hygiene, bathing, and homemaking. In a rehabilitation setting the occupational therapist retrains the brain injured person in self-care activities by the use of adaptive equipment or special techniques.

Adaptive equipment. Devices that allow a person to perform tasks that he previously could not carry out because of disability. Examples include button hooks, reachers, and stocking assists.

Affective behavior. The verbal and nonverbal patterns of behavior (facial expression, gestures, actions) associated with emotions, such as happiness, anger, distress, surprise, and pleasure. In a brain injured person emotional responses are often irrelevant and may not be appropriate to the situation.

Agitation. Excessive motor activity, which usually is nonproductive and repetitious and is often accompanied by shouting or loud complaining. Examples of agitated behavior include an inability to sit still, pacing, and pulling at clothes or other persons. Agitation is often associated with progress in recovery following brain injury.

Agnosia. Inability to recognize a sensory stimulus; may occur in any sensory modality.

Alertness. Refers to consciousness or wakefulness.

Ambulation. Walking.

Amnesia. Lack of memory for periods of time. There are several varieties:

Anterograde amnesia. Short term; inability to remember events beginning at the onset of the injury; essentially a severely decreased ability to learn.

Post-traumatic amnesia (PTA). The period of anterograde amnesia following a head injury; the patient is unable to store new information.

Retrograde amnesia. Long term; loss of memory for events preceding the injury.

Anomia. Inability to find the correct word. A person may seem to have the word "on the tip of the tongue" but simply cannot say the word.

Anoxia. An absence of oxygen supply to tissues.

Anxiety. A state of physical and psychological tension characterized by motor tension (inability to relax, jitteriness, trembling), physical symptoms (sweating, pounding heart, dry mouth, upset stomach, light-headedness, dizziness, increased pulse and respiration rates), apprehension, worry, fear, feeling of being "on edge," difficulty in falling asleep, interrupted sleep, and difficulty in concentrating.

Apathy. Lethargic or bland affect. A person exhibiting apathy may refuse to participate in or be disinterested in activities, and spends much of his time sitting or lying around. This lowered activity level is the result of impaired brain function and typically is not under the voluntary control of the brain injured person.

Aphasia. Impairment of some aspect of language; not due to defects in speech or hearing organs but to brain impairment; a total or partial loss of the ability to understand or to use words or symbols caused by brain injury, disease, or stroke; a language disturbance that affects comprehension, speaking, reading, writing, spelling, gesturing, and numerical calculating.

Apraxia. Inability to plan and execute a learned voluntary movement smoothly; not due to muscle weakness or failure to understand directions. For example, the person with apraxia has the strength and coordination to do a task and knows what he wants to do, but the brain is unable to program the movements necessary to complete the task.

Apraxia of speech. An impairment of speech caused by damage to the area of the brain responsible for planning orderly movements of the speech muscles; the partial or total inability to initiate or sequence speech sounds in the proper order even though the muscles of speech themselves may have adequate strength. For example, an attempt to say the word "banana" may result in the following types of errors: "falano," "banano," or "bananis." This disorder is easily recognized by the struggling and groping of the patient to control the speech muscles in an attempt to produce words.

Assessment. Measures used to systematically observe and record a person's language and cognitive and physical function. Assessment is employed to gain a complete understanding of the brain injured patient's strengths and weaknesses in order to determine areas of deficit and to plan a program for treatment.

Assistance. See Levels of assistance.

Ataxia. A lack of coordination that results in jerky, unsteady movements of the arms and legs.

Attention. The capacity for selective perception, for choosing the stimuli to perceive.

Augmentative communication devices and systems. An alternative communication device for nonverbal persons or a supplemental communication device to augment whatever verbal skills a person possesses. Examples are an alphabet board on which the individual spells out messages and a computer that can type out sentences entered by the patient, who merely focuses on the letters.

Automatic behavior. Actions that require little or no thought, effort, or planning. These actions are usually learned in childhood and are used frequently throughout life. Examples include reciting the alphabet or days of the week, tying shoelaces, and responding to social conventions (such as "How are you?").

Bagged. Use of a respirator bag to assist breathing.

Bed ex. An exercise program done on or near the bed.

Bed mobility. Movement in bed that includes rolling to each side and moving from sitting to lying and from lying to sitting positions.

Biofeedback. An external feedback system that allows a person to relearn how to move or relax muscles.

Bladder program. Since a physical disability often impairs bladder function, an indwelling (Foley) catheter is often put in place soon after the injury to allow for bladder drainage. This indwelling catheter may be removed, and a bladder program may be established to assist the person in regaining bladder control. This program may include fluid intake restrictions, a toileting schedule, periodic (intermittent) catheterization, and medications.

Body scheme. Refers to the knowledge of how one's body is put together and the relationships of body parts to each other. For example, a person with a body scheme disorder may not know that his hand is at the end of his arm and therefore may have trouble moving his hand in order to perform a functional task, such as putting on a shirt.

Bowel movement. In some persons disability causes an impairment in bowel function. In such cases the person's bowel patterns need to be re-established. This is done through a routine for bowel regulation, which incorporates diet, medication, and activity. This routine is established to reflect the prior habits of the individual as much as possible.

Carryover. Refers to the ability to retain newly learned skills or information and to apply them from situation to situation. In a rehabilitation setting this applies to voluntarily using strategies and techniques previously performed in therapy. These strategies and techniques have been taught to assist a brain injured person in compensating for areas of impairment.

Cerebrospinal fluid. The fluid within the subarachnoid space, the central canal of the spinal cord, and the four ventricles of the brain. This fluid cushions the brain and spinal cord from shock.

Closed head injury. Refers to a head injury in which the skull is not fractured or split.

Cognition (cognitive function). The ability to think and understand. Normal cognitive functioning involves intact skills of alertness; selective and gross attention to the environment; orientation to time, person, or place; concentration; memory; knowledge; insight; emotional control; judgment; problem solving; language; and empathy and the ability to anticipate the consequences of behavior. One or all of these cognitive skills may be affected in a brain injured person and may interfere with learning. The impairment of these cognitive skills often may be upsetting to family members.

Cognitive flexibility. The ability to shift one's cognitive or perceptual set.

Coma. A state of unconsciousness from which a person cannot be aroused, even by powerful stimuli.

Community education. A program designed to teach brain injured persons and their families about resources found in the community and how to use them, including recreation programs, transportation services, and support organizations. Community education also addresses the rights of the disabled person as well as the accessibility issues.

Comprehension. The ability to process language of varying complexity, relating that information to past experiences and acting upon it appropriately; comprehension is determined by the patient's behavior.

Concrete thinking. Difficulty in forming abstract concepts, in speculating about what might be, and in grouping similar things into categories.

Concussion. Refers to a loss of consciousness following an injury to the head, with recovery in a short while. A concussion is caused by a sudden jar or shock to the brain.

Confabulation. Verbalization about people, places, and events with no basis in reality; may be detailed and delivered with apparent confidence by the patient. This disturbance is related to the person's inability to interpret and integrate events and accompanies confusion and memory disturbances. Often these stories reflect the person's effort to make sense of the environment. Confabulation differs from lying in that the individual actually believes what he is reporting and is not attempting to deceive.

Confusion. Disturbances in the ability to accurately interpret or make sense of environmental events. The person who is confused may become agitated or verbally aggressive because he is unable to understand where he is and is unable to recognize individuals in the environment or the reasons for pain or discomfort. The language of the individual who is confused may seem unorganized, disconnected, or meaningless to the listener. The responses of the brain injured person may have nothing to do with the topic of conversation.

Constructional apraxia. Inability to assemble, build, draw, or copy accurately; not due to apraxia of single movements.

Contracture. Loss of flexibility (range of motion) in a joint due to changes in a joint, tendon, or ligament.

Contrecoup. A term referring to an injury occurring in a part of the brain opposite the point of impact. This "contrecoup" injury is caused by changes in pressure, which travel through the brain.

Contusion. A bruising (in this case, of the brain), which causes tissue damage and bleeding.

Decubitus ulcer. Pressure sore.

Depression. A significant persistent change in mood characterized by the patient's description of his mood as sad, blue, hopeless, low, "down in the dumps," or irritable. Depression often is accompanied by a loss of interest or pleasure in most or all of the patient's usual activities or pastimes. A depressed individual may complain of loss of energy, feelings of inadequacy or worthlessness, and difficulty in concentrating and often expresses thoughts of suicide or death. These symptoms are often accompanied by social withdrawal, decreased effectiveness in activities, tearfulness, pessimism, and sleep disorders. Even though most individuals have a sense of what it means to feel depressed, the actual diagnosis of depression is complicated. Medical complications, medications, or environmental factors often result in symptoms that imitate those of depression.

Diaphoresis. Excessive sweating.

Diffuse involvement. An injury that impairs the functioning of large areas of brain tissue.

Discrimination. The ability to discern fine differences among stimuli, whether visual, auditory, tactile, or other types.

Disinhibition. Refers to an impairment in the ability to control one's own behavior, resulting in occasional or frequent displays of socially inappropriate behavior, decreased impulse control, and difficulty in the control of emotions.

Dressings. Protective coverings for wounds.

Dysarthria. Difficulty with pronunciation; due to weakness or poor coordination of muscles of the lips, tongue, and jaw. Speech may sound slurred, slowed, distorted, weak, and nasal. Speech content is unaffected.

Dyscalculia. Impaired ability to do arithmetic computation; may relate to a variety of more basic disorders such as confusion or deficits in perception, spatial skills, and sequencing; sometimes referred to as acalculia, which is technically a total inability to do arithmetic.

Dysgraphia. Impaired ability to write; not due to motor impairment; also referred to as "agraphia," which is technically a total inability to write.

Dyslexia. Impaired ability to read.

Dysphagia. A disturbance in the ability to swallow either solid foods or liquids. Problems interfering with normal swallowing may occur at any point from the mouth to the stomach. Swallowing problems may result from muscular disturbances, neurological damage, or loss of sensation. Decreased alertness may also affect normal swallowing in that a person may be unaware of food in his mouth.

Edema. Swelling caused by extra water in the soft tissues.

Electroencephalography (EEG). A test that measures the electrical activity of the brain.

Emesis. Vomiting.

Euphoria. An exaggerated feeling of well-being; mild elation.

Equipment (assistive devices). Devices needed to increase independence. Examples include braces, wheelchairs, bathroom equipment, and walking aids. Such equipment is individually designed to meet a particular patient's needs.

Ex (exercise). This usually denotes a mat program used for physical therapy. Time also may be spent doing advanced transfer training, family teaching, and equipment evaluation.

Executive functions. Planning, prioritizing, sequencing, self-monitoring, self-correcting, inhibiting, initiating, controlling, or altering behavior.

Evoked cerebral response test. A test used to measure the brain's response time to a visual, auditory, or tactile (somatosensory) stimulus.

Field cut. See Hemianopsia.

Finger agnosia. Inability to determine which finger is being stimulated by touch alone.

Flaccidity. Lack of muscle tone, resulting in inability to perform a movement.

Foley catheter. An indwelling catheter used to provide drainage of urine when bladder function is impaired.

Foot drop. Results from lack of movement or manipulation; the foot drops downward and remains in that position; treated by corrective footwear and manipulation.

Functional. Refers to the ability to accomplish a task using any means available, e.g., adaptive equipment and compensation techniques.

Goal directed, purposeful behavior. Actions directed toward the accomplishment of specific objectives or the fulfillment of intention or desire. Such behavior appears to be organized, controlled, and efficient.

Group home. A closely supervised living situation for disabled individuals that focuses on the development of self-help skills to prepare individuals for semi-independent or independent living.

Hematoma. A localized collection of blood in an organ, space, or tissue. In brain injury, three types of hematomas are common: subdural, epidural, and intracerebral.

Hemianopsia. Blindness of one half of the field of vision caused by brain damage. The term does not refer to blindness in one eye; rather it indicates blindness of one half of each (either side) and normal vision in the other half of each eye.

Hemorrhage. The escape of blood from a ruptured vessel.

Higher cognitive functions. Usually refers to judgment, abstraction, problem solving, and planning.

Hoyer® lift. Equipment used to transfer a person safely to and from the bed to a wheelchair and vice versa.

Hypoxia. A decrease in the oxygen supply to tissues.

Hydrocephalus. Excess accumulation of cerebrospinal fluid, causing increased intra-cranial pressure.

Hydrotherapy. Treatment using water as a means of promoting relaxation and healing, increasing flexibility, and decreasing pain. Such treatment may involve the use of a variety of water tanks, including Hubbard tanks, walking tanks, whirlpools, and lowboys.

Impairment. A decrease in the strength or quality of a function because of sickness or injury.

Imperception, inattention, suppression, extinction. All these terms refer to a failure to perceive stimulation on one side of the body when both sides are being stimulated simultaneously (double simultaneous stimulation); not due to a primary sensory deficit such as deafness, blindness, or dysesthesia (numbness); appears to be an attentional deficit; is less severe than neglect and may occur in a patient recovering from neglect.

Intermediate care facility. A facility providing personal care to individuals who demonstrate an intermediate degree of physical or social dependency. Minimal medical nursing care is provided. The emphasis is on a structured supportive care system with minimal physical assistance in meeting daily living needs.

Intracerebral. Refers to the inside of the brain itself.

Intracranial. Refers to the cavity inside the skull that contains the brain.

Isolation. Precautions taken to protect the brain injured person and others, usually from the spread of infection.

Judgment. The ability to make appropriate decisions based upon available information and expected consequences; the ability to effectively manage vocational choices, personal finances, and social situations and to make day to day living decisions that most of us take for granted.

Lack of insight and denial. Lack of awareness of problems that warrant change. A person may completely deny the existence of a disability because he is unaware of existing cognitive problems. When this condition persists, it may seriously interfere with a person's ability to return to a previous life style.

Language. Usually refers to the ability to enter new information into long term memory; any means of expressing or communicating thought and feelings; can include hand gestures and facial expression as well as speech, writing, and the ability to use numbers. Language also refers to the structure (grammar) and meaning (semantics) of thoughts and feelings and their expression. A brain injury or stroke may disrupt thought processes and result in confused or disturbed language expression.

Levels of assistance:

Dependent. The brain injured person who makes no voluntary effort to assist.

Maximal assistance. The brain injured person participates minimally, and another person performs most of the activity.

Moderate assistance. The brain injured person and another person participate about equally in performance of the activity.

Constant minimal assistance. The brain injured person performs most of the activity, and another person assists minimally but constantly.

Occasional minimal cuing. The brain injured person performs most of the activity, and another person provides minimal assistance occasionally.

Verbal cues. The brain injured person requires observation by another person and verbal cues to perform the activity in order to avoid the need for physical assistance or to avoid a potential safety hazard.

Supervision. The brain injured person requires observation by another person to insure consistently safe performance of the activity.

Independent. The brain injured person requires no assistance or supervision to perform the activity.

Lightening up. The gradual awakening from a coma.

Long term memory. See under Memory.

Manual dexterity. The ability to coordinate one's hands to accomplish basic specific tasks, e.g., typing and dialing a telephone.

Medical assistance. Refers to medical insurance provided by the state or federal government for persons who meet certain medical or financial eligibility standards. Usually this means that the individual or his family has been divested of virtually all money and property to be eligible.

Memory. Recording of new information; many types of memory are distinguished depending on the person's theoretical orientation. Some of the more common are:

Delayed recall. Recall of material after a delay, often with intervening material being introduced to prevent active rehearsal.

Episodic memory. Memory for continuing events in a person's life; more easily impaired than semantic memory, perhaps because rehearsal or repetition tends to be minimal.

Immediate recall. Immediate repetition of information given by the examiner.

Long term memory. More permanent storage of the memory trace; events that have occurred prior to an injury. For example, previous employment, family members, and residential history represent long term memory events. This type of past information is typically partially or wholly preserved in many brain injured individuals.

Nonverbal memory. Memory for figures, spatial relationships; assumed to be based in the deep structures of the right temporal lobe.

Registration. A very brief sensory-memory function by which information enters the memory system; it is then entered into short term memory or decays and is lost; very resistant to impairment.

Short term memory. Working memory with a limited capacity; the ability to remember momentary events. Its contents are in conscious awareness; lasts 30 seconds to several minutes. Short term memory loss may range from the occasional forgetting of names to a total loss of memory for events after only a few minutes. Short term memory problems are the most common memory impairments exhibited by brain injured persons.

Verbal memory. Memory for verbal information; assumed to reflect functioning of the deep structures of the left temporal lobe.

Modalities. A general term used to describe treatments using heat, cold, light, and water. These treatments are commonly used to help reduce pain, increase functional movement, reduce contractures, and promote healing, for example. They are prescribed by a physician on the basis of the individual's needs. Examples of modalities are ultraviolet, ultrasound, hot packs, and functional electrical stimulation.

Motor control. The ability to selectively contract or relax a muscle or group of muscles at will.

Muscle tone. The amount of tension (continuous contraction) in a muscle at rest. The quality or quantity of muscle tone affects the efficiency of voluntary muscle contraction. For example, when a person has low muscle tone, his endurance will be less and he will react less to a given stimulus. Therapy for abnormal muscle tone is designed to normalize tone by either decreasing spasticity (high muscle tone) to facilitate movement or, in the case of low muscle tone, improving tone to allow more ease of movement.

Neglect. Severe lack of awareness of the side of space contralateral to a brain lesion; may occur in any sensory modality; more pronounced than imperception.

Neuropsychological evaluation. An assessment using psychological tests, interviews, and behavioral observation to determine a person's cognitive, emotional, and behavioral state, with emphasis on deficiencies of intellect, personality, and behavior as outcomes of brain injury. Such assessment attempts to determine brain-behavior relationships, location of injuries, and brain systems involved.

Oral-motor function. Movement of the lips, tongues, and soft palate.

Orientation. Reality-based information about the world, e.g., who one is, where one is, whom one is talking to, and what day it is.

Organic personality syndrome. A change in personality marked by impaired judgment and a loss of control over emotions, impulses, and behavior. "Organic" personality changes result from a specific physical cause (e.g., brain injury). A person with the organic personality syndrome may exhibit sudden temper outbursts, sudden crying spells, apathy, indifference, loss of initiative, suspiciousness, and anxiety, as well as other behavioral or emotional difficulties.

Paraphrasia. Use of incorrect words or word combinations.

Perception. Integration of sensory impressions into psychologically meaningful data.

Perseveration. Meaningless repetition of a verbal or motor response, or repetition of answers that are not related to successive questions asked.

Posey. A safety harness used to prevent falls.

Positioning. Placing a person in a position such that muscle and joint flexibility is preserved and skin breakdown is prevented. Positioning is especially important for persons with the potential for contractures or limited mobility. A variety of positions are needed for each individual. A person's position must be changed at prescribed intervals to obtain maximal benefit.

Pressure sores. Also called decubitus ulcers. Open sores due to prolonged pressure and immobility that often appear on the coccyx, sacrum, ankles, and elbows. Major methods of pressure sore prevention include good nutrition, correct positioning, frequent turning when in bed, and weight shifting when in a wheelchair.

Problem solving. The ability to integrate and evaluate the various parts of a situation and to anticipate possible consequences in order to arrive at a productive conclusion.

Proprioception. Perception of the position of one's limbs in space. For example, a person with proprioceptive loss may be unaware that his arm has fallen off the armrest and is dangling outside the wheelchair.

Prosody. The inflections and intonations of speech.

Purposeful-nonpurposeful movement. As the terms imply, purposeful movement is movement with an intended goal. Nonpurposeful movement is movement without an apparent goal.

Range of motion. Exercises specifically directed to movement of joints that may atrophy from disuse.

    Active range of motion. The amount of motion at a given joint achieved by a person using his own muscle strength to move the joint.

    Passive range of motion. The amount of motion at a given joint when the joint is moved by another person or by another functioning limb of the brain injured individual.

Right sided neglect. See Unilateral neglect.

Seizure, seizure disorder. A disturbance in the electrical-chemical activity of the brain due to nerve cell damage or electrolyte imbalance. After a brain injury, scar tissue in the brain may lead to reduced seizure tolerance (also known as a seizure disorder or post-traumatic epilepsy). Seizures are usually common during the first two years after injury and usually decrease in frequency as time goes on. Alcohol consumption by a seizure prone person can increase his risk of having a seizure.

Self-monitoring. Awareness of one's behavior and the accuracy or appropriateness of one's performance; usually automatic and continuing.

Sensation. Sensory stimulation, passively received; involves no processing or manipulation of sensory information.

Sequencing skills. The ability to order elements correctly; may be motor (sequencing body movements smoothly) or linguistic (sequencing words appropriately into sentences) or may involve keeping track of the correct order of stimuli.

Serial casting. A technique used to reduce contractures and to control hypertonicity in and around a joint, usually the ankles and wrists. It involves the use of a series of plaster casts, which are applied to the area every seven to 10 days. When the cast is changed, the joint should be recasted in an improved position. The casting is usually continued until a functional position is obtained.

Sheltered workshop. Work oriented rehabilitation facility with a controlled environment. Such a workshop employs disabled people and provides work experience that may assist the individual in progressing toward a productive vocational status.

Short term memory. See under Memory.

Skilled care facility. A facility in which nursing services, therapy services, and other sources of physical support are provided to individuals with physical or cognitive limitations. An example of a skilled care facility is a nursing home.

Sling. An external device applied to the arm to provide support and positioning of a weakened extremity.

Social interaction-socialization. Socialization refers to the skills needed to participate in the social situations that are part of living. Therapeutic recreation assists a brain injured individual in building such needed social skills. In order to do this, the therapeutic recreation specialist evaluates how the person interacts with other people. Does the person relate better with individuals or with a group? Will the person initiate a conversation with some, or does he always need to have conversation directed at him? Does the person withdraw from others, or does he seek to be with other people? On the basis of answers to such questions the recreation specialist works with the individual to enhance social skills.

Social security disability. Refers to monthly income granted to persons who have paid into the Social Security system and are confirmed disabled and unable to work for at least one year. This coverage also provides health insurance through the Medicare program if the disability continues beyond two years.

Spasms. Involuntary muscle contractions resulting from excessive muscle tone caused by an interruption of controlling impulses in the brain and spinal cord.

Spasticity. An uncontrolled increase in muscle tone at rest or during movement. Depending on its degree, spasticity may cause difficulty in movement or coordination. Spasticity tends to occur in patterns. For example, when a person raises his shoulders, his elbow may automatically bend and his hand closes. Such patterns of spasticity can make functional living activities difficult (e.g., eating, personal hygiene).

Spatial relations. Related to visual perception, spatial relations ability is the ability to understand the relationships of objects in space and of objects to each other.

Speech. Oral expression of language.

Splint. An external device applied to an extremity to provide positioning to help prevent or correct contractures.

Spontaneous recovery. Behavioral outcome of the natural healing process of the nervous system.

Stimulus-stimuli. Anything causing or intending to cause a response. For example, calling out a person's name and holding a person's hands are both stimuli.

Suction machine. Used to remove secretions from oral or nasal passages.

Supplemental security income (SSI). Refers to a federal income maintenance program for the aged, blind, and disabled who have limited income and resources; administered through the Social Security Administration. People who receive supplemental security income generally receive Medical Assistance as well.

Team conference (staffing). A periodic meeting of a patient's rehabilitation team. At the team conference the patient's progress, rehabilitation goals, and estimated length of stay are discussed and documented. Families are periodically contacted by either the patient's program manager or his psychologist to discuss details of the topics discussed at these conferences.

Tilt table. A table that has the capacity to raise and lower a person from the horizontal to the vertical position and vice versa. It is used to stretch heel cords or to increase standing tolerance in those who have not been in an upright position for an extended period of time.

Transfers. Basic transers include movement to and from a bed and chair. Advanced transfers refer to movement to and from a toilet, car, tub or shower, or floor.

Trunk. The region of the body from the shoulder to the pelvis.

Trunk control. The ability of a person to maintain proper alignment of the head, neck, and pelvis; to bring the trunk back into alignment after displacement; and to move the trunk at will (for example, to twist).

Treatment. Individual or group therapy designed to improve problem areas identified in the team's assessment.

Tube feeding. Nutritional feedings administered through a gastrostomy tube (a permanent or semipermanent tube placed in the stomach) or a nasogastric tube (a permanent or semipermanent tube placed in the pharynx or esophagus) when swallowing is impaired.

Unilateral neglect (hemineglect, hemiattention). The inability to interpret and use sensation and information from one half of the body or environment.

Urinary tract infection. A bacterial infection in the urinary tract (e.g., bladder infection).

Videofluoroscopy. An examination designed to detect any difficulties a person may have in swallowing in order that appropriate therapeutic measures may be taken.

Visual perception. The brain's ability to organize and interpet what is being seen so that one can act in response. For example, visual perception gives a person the ability to see a footstool, judge its size and shape, judge one's distance from it, and walk around it rather than bumping into it. Visual perceptual impairment may cause a person to have difficulty in dressing because he is unable to distinguish a shirt from a pair of slacks or to identify a shirt's right sleeve from the left or the top of the shirt from the bottom.

Vocational counseling. The process of assisting the disabled person to understand his vocational assets and liabilities and of providing occupational information to help him choose an occupation suitable for his interests and abilities.

Voice, voice function. The sound produced by a vibration of the vocal cords. A brain injury or stroke may cause paralysis, weakness, or discoordination of vocal cord movement, resulting in hoarseness, breathiness, reduced volume, changes in pitch, monotone, or absence of voice.

Voiding. Urinating.

BIBLIOGRAPHY

Pamphlets and Booklets

The Brain Injury Rehabilitation Programs at St. Lawrence Rehabilitation Center. Lawrenceville, NJ.

DeBoskey D, Morin K: A "How to Handle" Manual for Families of the Brain Injured. Tampa, Fl, Hillsborough County Hospital Authority Printing and Graphic Services, 1985.

Facilitator Job Description. Jenkintown, PA: Crossroads Healthcare Services, Inc.

Hawley LA: A Family Guide to the Rehabilitation of the Severely Head-Injured Patient: Head Injury Services of the Brown Schools. Healthcare International Inc., 1984.

Head Trauma Family Guide. Camden, NJ: Lourdes Regional Rehabilitation Center.

Help for the Head Injured and their Families. West Chester, PA: Pennsylvania Association of the NHIF.

Lake Erie Institute of Rehabilitation: Departmental Services Booklet. Camp Hill, PA: Rehabilitation Hospital Services Corp.

Lake Erie Institute of Rehabilitation: Patient/Family Booklet. Camp Hill, PA: Rehabilitation Hospital Services Corp.

Owen S, Toomin H, Taylor LP: Biofeedback in Neuromuscular Re-education. Biofeedback Research Institute, 1975.

Rehab Quarterly. Williamsport, PA: The Williamsport Hospital.

Sensory Integration — Information for Parents. Albany, CA: Bay Area Association for Sensory Integration.

Update Rehab. Langhorne, PA: Saint Mary Hospital, 1986.

Tower System: Evaluator's Manual, I.C.D. Rehabilitation and Research Center, NY, 1967.

Valpar Component Work Sample Series. Valpar Corporation, Tucson, AZ, 1974-1977.

Journals

Bruckner FE, Randle APH: Return to work after severe head injuries. Rheum Phys Med 11:344-348, 1972.

Campbell MK (Ed): Topics in Acute Care and Rehabilitation 1(1), Rockville, Md, Aspen Publications, July 1986.

Cognitive Rehabilitation, 3(4), 1985.

Connecticut Health Bulletin, 96(4), 1982.

Dresser AC, et al.: Gainful employment following head injury. Arch Neurol 29:111-116, 1973.

Heaton RK, Chelune GJ, Lehman RAW: Using neuropyschological and personality tests to assess the likelihood of patient employment. J Nerv Ment Disor 166:408-416, 1978.

Jennett B, Bond M: Assessment of outcome after severe brain damage. Lancet, 1975, p 480.

Kwentus J: Psychiatric Complications of Closed Head Trauma. Psychosomatics 26(2): 8-17.

Newman OS, Heatch RK, Lehman RAW: Neurological and MMP correlates of patients' future employment characteristics. Percept Motor Skills 46:635-642, 1978.

Rappaport M, et al.: Disability rating scale for severe head trauma: Coma to community. Arch Phys Med Rehabil 63 (March): 1982.

Books

Ayres AJ: Sensory Integration and the Child. Los Angeles, CA, Western Psychological Services, 1979.

Ayres AJ: Sensory Integration and Learning Disorders. Los Angeles, CA, Western Psychological Services, 1980.

Bobath B: Abnormal Postural Reflex Activity Caused by Brain Lesions. Ed. 2. William Heinemann Medical Books, 1971.

Bobath B: Adult Hemiplegia: Evaluation and Treatment. Ed 2. London, William Heinemann Medical Books, 1978.

Brain L, Walton N: Brain Diseases of the Nervous System. Ed 7. New York, Oxford University Press, 1969.

Carr J, Shepherd R: Motor Relearning Programme for Stroke. Rockville, MD, Aspen Publications, 1983.

Davies PM: Steps to Follow. Berlin, Springer Verlag, 1985.

Jennett B: An Introducction to neurosurgery. Ed 3. London, William Heinemann Medical Books, 1977.

Rosenthal M, et al.: Rehabilitation of the Head Injured Adult. Philadelphia, F. A. Davis Company, 1983.

Siev E, Freishtat B, Zoltan B: Perceptual and Cognitive Dysfunction in the Adult Stroke Patient. Thorofare, NJ: Slack, Inc., 1986.

White R: Abnormal Psychology. New York: Ronald Press Co., 1956.

Personal Interviews

Bryn Mawr Rahabilitation Center, Malvern, PA.
Cooper Hospital/University Medical Center, Camden, NJ.
Moss Rehabilitation Center, Philadelphia, PA.
National Head Injury Association, Inc., Framingham, MA
New Jersey Chapter of the National Head Injury Association, Inc., NJ.
Pennsylvania Chapter of the National Head Injury Association, Inc., PA.
Our Lady of Lourdes Hospital, Camden, NJ.
REACH, Manor Healthcare Corp., Silver Spring, MD.
St. Lawrence Rehabilitation Center, Lawrenceville, NJ.
Meadowbrook Neurologic Care Center, 340 Northlake Drive, San Jose, CA 95117
Tangrum Ranch, San Marcos, Texas
Dr. H. Carberry, Our Lady of Lourdes Hospital, Rehabilitation Division, Camden, NJ.
Dr. Keating, Moss Rehabilitation Center, Philadelphia, PA.
Dr. Willard-Mack, St. Lawrence Rehabilitation Center, Lawrenceville, NJ.

DATE DUE